FACEWORKS

The
COMPLETE FACELIFT
Workout

Elaine Bartlett

faceexerciseguru.com

Text, Logo and Illustrations © 2013 Elaine Bartlett
Studio Photography ©2013 Immortaleye Photography Ltd.
All exercise photos are of Elaine at the age of 53
The rights of Elaine Bartlett to be identified as author of this work ,and as owner of the Faceworks Face Exercise program has been asserted in accordance with the Copyright, Designs and Patents Act, 1998.

ISBN 978-1-8380230-0-3

All rights reserved. No part of this publication may be reproduced, stored in a retrieval system, or transmitted in any form or by any means, electronic, mechanical, photocopied, recorded or otherwise, without the prior written permission of the author.

Disclaimer

As with any new exercise program, it is advisable that you check with your GP to make sure the Faceworks exercises are suitable for you before beginning the program, even if you consider yourself to be fully fit.
Please bear in mind this book is not intended to be a substitute for medical advice or treatment from your doctor or any other medical specialist. Neither the publisher or author accept any responsibility for any legal or medical liability or other consequences , which may arise directly or indirectly as a consequence from any use or misuse of the information contained in this book.

To my wonderful and indestructible family

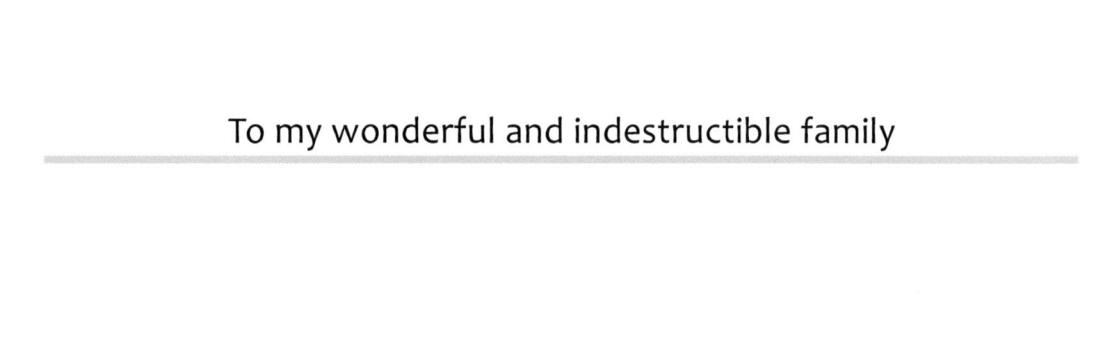

Contents

Introduction 1

But Does it Really Work? 3

    Before and after photos 6

The Basics for Fabulous Faces 11

Part One 13

About You 15

    What Would You Like to Change? 15

    How You Look Now 18

    Your Wish List 20

Part Two 23

    Workout Videos 24

The Face Exercises 25

    How to Get Your Facelift 25

    Faceworks Diary 28

Results Timeline 34

    Two Weeks 34

    One Month 34

    Two Months 35

    Three Months 35

    Three Months Plus 36

Exercise 1: Facial Warm-up 40

Exercise 2: Mouth Shaper One 42

Exercise 3: Mouth Shaper Two 44

Exercise 4: Lip Builder 46

Exercise 5: Eyebrow Lift 49

Exercise 6: Cheek Toner One 52

    Creating Killer Cheekbones with the Cheek Toners 56

Exercise 8: Eye Toner Two 60

Exercise 9: Chin and Jaw Toner 62

Exercise 10: Cheek Toner Two 65

Exercise 11: Mouth Area Shaper 68

Exercise 12: Face Finisher 70

Relaxing Massage 73

Questions and Problems 76

The Express Workout 81

    The Instant Boosters: Your Secret Weapon 82

The Mini Workouts 83

Quick List 1: Effects and Results 85

Quick List 2: Your Personal Face Savers 88

Part Three 91

The Science of Facial Exercise 93

    The Right Facial Balance 93

    Your Facial Muscles 94

    Diagram 1: Superficial and Deep Facial Muscle Layers 94

    Diagram 2: Superficial Facial Muscle Layer, Lateral View 95

    Diagram 3: Deep Facial Muscle Layer, Lateral View 96

    How Exercise Rebuilds Your Facial Muscles 98

    Anatomy of the Skin 99

    How Facial Exercise Transforms Your Skin 100

A Note on Cosmetic Surgery	101
The Ageing Face	102
Ageing Timeline	104
The Development of Faceworks	106
Postscript	109
Glossary of Terms	110
Acknowledgements	113
Bibliography and Resources	114

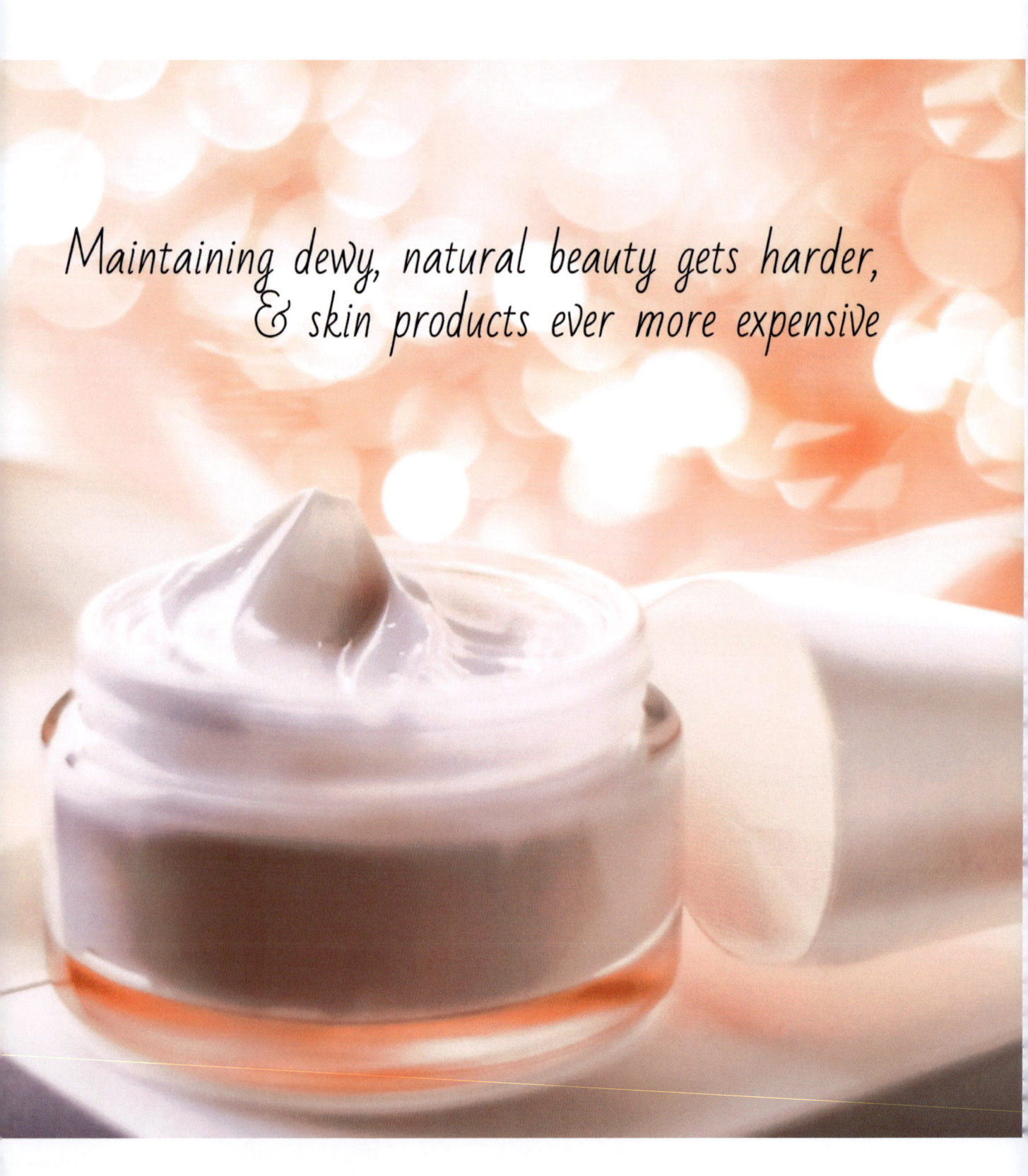

Introduction

On the days when you feel fantastic about how you look, life is wonderful. If by some miracle of science it were possible to bottle that precise feel-good emotion, it would be a million pound best seller. But as age increases; maintaining that dewy and natural beauty gets harder, skin products get ever more expensive and those 'feel good days' dwindle away.

The desire to stay looking good keeps us spending. The need to age well (or look younger) drives a multi-billion pound industry to satisfy the demand for ever-more sophisticated skincare products. But the truth is that no product applied to the skin can solve the problem completely, because they don't reach the layers where new cells are made. Skin products are beneficial for the top layers of the dermis but they don't reach deep enough into the skin or the supporting tissues below. And the **real** secret to ageing well lies here.

Your body has the ability to regenerate itself. It's time to use it.

Therapy Background
I belatedly trained in alternative therapies my late 30s, qualifying as a Reiki Master and Kinesiologist in 2001 at the age of 40. Perhaps as a result of the 'late entry' into therapies, advising clients on ways to maximise their health potential sparked an interest in anti-ageing. After developing Faceworks and having it accepted as a Registered Therapy, the focus of my practice gradually changed from seeing clients for general health optimising to purely anti-ageing.

The reality of face exercises was astonishing: I discovered that dramatic changes were possible, so good in fact that people thought I had gone 'under the knife'. Incidentally, I have nothing against cosmetic surgery. It is just that with Faceworks I don't feel I need to explore having any. The testimonials from people who use the program are often similar in that their friends and family often assume the changes are due to surgery.

Previous to my career change, I studied naturopathic methods of healing and cleansing the body with renowned herbalist Kitty Campion. Under Kitty's expert guidance, I cured the ill health that had persisted through my late 20s and 30s. I continue to use my therapies and naturopathic methods to maintain my own and my family's health. Faceworks is the icing on the cake.

Qualifications:

- Foundation Course: the Kinesiology Association (Registered Charity No. 299306)
- Advanced Course in Systematic Kinesiology: John Logue College of Professional Kinesiology
- ITEC Anatomy and Physiology Diploma, with Credits
- KA Nutritional Certificate
- Usui Reiki I, Usui Reiki II and Usui Reiki Master
- Tsuboki Japanese Face Massage
- Certificate in Facial Treatments and Face Massage

But Does it Really Work?

This book is for people who want to age well and look great forever

If you want to rejuvenate how you look and stop looking old, this book will bring back the face you thought you'd lost. There's no reason to give in to deep wrinkles, sagging, or other signs of age that are appearing on your face. Really, there isn't. Beautiful skin and a toned and lifted face are achievable naturally with face exercises, and the exercises are proven to:

- Reduce wrinkles and lines
- Lift and firm facial skin
- Reshape and rejuvenate the whole face
- Lift sagging and shapeless facial contours
- Enhance and lift the eyebrows, erase frown furrows
- Lift, smooth and rejuvenate the eye area
- Sculpt and re-contour the cheeks
- Erase nasolabial folds and furrows
- Plump the lips and tone up the mouth area
- Neaten and firm the jawline
- Tone and reduce double chins

Rejuvenating the facial muscles brings so many benefits to the structure and appearance of the face, both now and in the future. The exercises actively slow down new signs of ageing from spreading. A toned, firm face doesn't sag. Skin that's kept in good condition by optimum blood flow looks younger because it glows. Which means it's possible to stay looking great for the rest of your life.

All kinds of people use the exercises; including beauty professionals, fitness instructors, doctors and surgeons:

> *"As a member of the general public as well as a makeup artist I can tell you that I've not only had very good results personally but my clients have benefited for it greatly. I'd recommend it for anybody!"*
> *Trisha, Canada*

So if this works, I never need to look old again?
It does work and no, you won't. You'll never dread your holiday photos again. Each sign of facial ageing has been matched with an exercise to restore that precise area. You will still look like 'you', but on a good day; with smooth, healthy skin and a firm face. People will ask if you've had 'work' done, they'll tell you how great you look, though they'll never guess how you're doing it.

How much younger?
If you do all the exercises in the Complete Workout, you can expect to look 7-10 years younger than you do now. Twelve years of feedback show some people achieve quite a bit more than that. People regularly mistake me for being 10-12 years younger and I've had a good few jaw-drops when the truth comes out. Be prepared to need a big stick to fight off admirers: or maybe just enjoy the attention!

Do face exercises really work?
Yes, they do. The exercise photos are all of me in my 50s: surgery-free. (I've never had fillers or Botox either). Facial muscles tone up just the same as body muscles – but, and here's the BIG secret - facial muscles are attached to the base layers of the skin: the dermis. If they weren't, you wouldn't be able to move your face, or talk, laugh, or kiss. So when you tone and lift facial muscles with exercise, the skin lifts and tightens too.

What is Faceworks?
Faceworks is scientifically developed and the only face exercise program to gain approval as a Professional Registered Therapy. The program is designed to be easy and gives results that will minimise the signs of aging for life. Faceworks has lifted and transformed my tired and drooping face and it can lift and transform yours, too.

How long does it take to do?
You choose how much you want to do, depending on the results you want. There are 12 multi-tasking exercises in total, all cleverly designed to work together, or individually. The Complete Workout takes 30 minutes and gives a complete facelift. The Express Workout takes 15 minutes, and the Mini Workouts exercise one area of the face in 10 minutes.

How long does it take to get results?
The first results are noticeable by about 10 days, sometimes sooner. Many reviews come from people who are amazed by the changes in the first month to 6 weeks. A complete facelift takes approximately 12 weeks, depending on how much sagging is present, and

improvements are constant throughout this time. When you're happy with how you look, the 3-4 times a week maintenance program keeps you looking great indefinitely.

How much will Faceworks change my face?
The exercises gently reshape the face. The changes enhance your own beauty rather than changing the bone structure. The exercises can't alter your face as drastically as surgery can, for example, they won't increase the size of your jaw or make your nose smaller.

Won't face exercises cause wrinkles?
Faceworks won't. Never mind what you've heard. The exercises are carefully designed not to stretch the skin or add to lines and wrinkles already there. As the exercises take effect, the skin plumps and improves so that deep lines, wrinkles and folds smooth out.

Isn't it all too good to be true?
If someone asks me this, I tell them how old I am, and watch for the sideways look of disbelief. I look better now at nearly 60 than I did at 45.

Faceworks has been taught to clients in my therapy practice, to people in shops and in business meetings, to thousands of people via the videos online; and I still use the exercises to keep my own face toned and lifted. Yet when I was in my early 40's, I despaired of ever looking young again.

Despite trying every 'miracle' cream within my budget, I looked old: my face was slowly turning into my mother's. I wanted my young face back: the one that had seen me through fun, love and laughter, had acquired a husband, and had enjoyed the occasional second glance.

Now I have the face I desperately wanted back, without surgery, Botox, or fillers. It's no exaggeration to say that the exercises have transformed my confidence and personal happiness. I am not afraid of aging because I know I can continue to look healthy and fabulous in the years to come. It's a great feeling to have.

What *doesn't* Faceworks do?
Faceworks won't change your bone structure or drastically alter your face. Radical changes aren't possible with facial exercise: it is a much gentler and more natural approach than surgery. The exercises won't over-build or bulk up your facial muscles like a body-builder or increase the size of your features, because facial muscles rebuild within their natural ability.

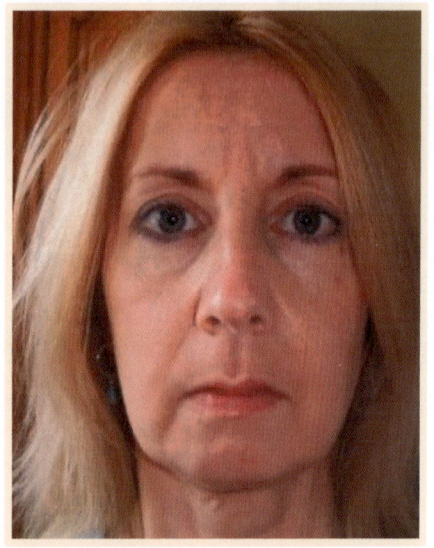

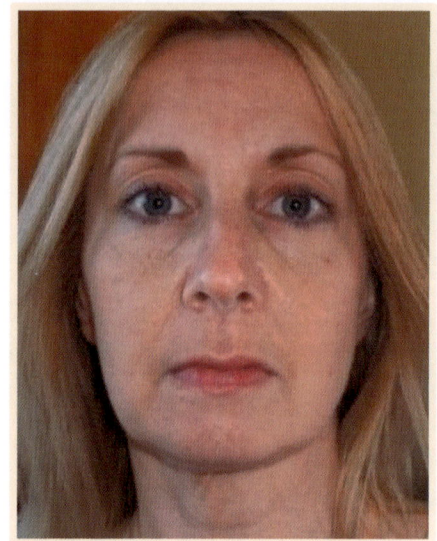

Age 45

Before Faceworks

July 2006

Exercise Schedule: None

I was happy in this photo: you'd never guess! Generally 'tired' appearance, with uneven looking and dull skin, lines between very low brows, sagging eyelids, hollows under the eyes, flat cheeks, sagging lower cheeks and deep 'marionette' folds each side of my mouth. My jawline is droopy and my neck has slack skin at the front. No wonder my children said I looked cross all the time!

Age 45

After 4 weeks

August 2006

Exercise schedule: the Complete Workout 5 times per week.

The skin is brighter and smoother, brows are lifted with reduced lines in between and eyes are brighter. Under-eye hollows are a little reduced and the cheeks are plumped, which has lifted the lower cheeks and the folds around my mouth. The lower face looks neater with less sagging at the jawline. What's surprising is my nose is less 'lumpy' across the top.

Before and after photos over 13 years of Faceworks

These 4 photos above were taken in natural daylight – there's no studio lighting, special effects or editing such as Photoshop. If you'd met me on the day these were taken this is genuinely how I would look.

Make-up this page, left and right photos: Nivea Tinted Moisturiser in Light, Powder: unknown, Bourjois blusher: Fraicher de Rose, L'Oreal eyeliner: Blue Denim, Mascara: Max Factor Masterpiece Max.

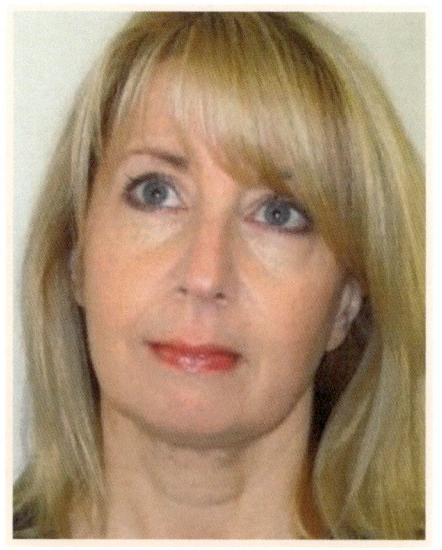 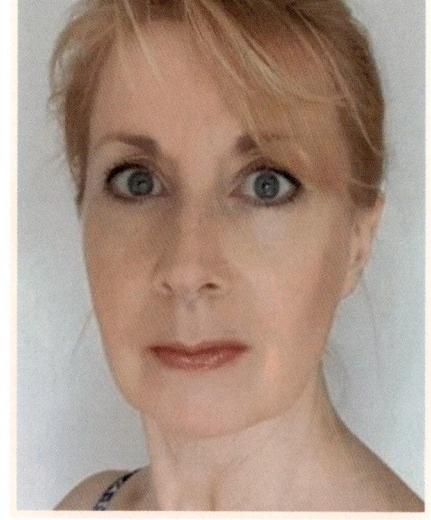

Age 50
After 6 years

November 2011

Exercise Schedule: the Complete Workout 3-4 times per week.
Skin look resilient and healthy. The brows and eyes are defined and the bridge and top of the nose is neater. The shape of my face is more contoured over the cheeks as the muscles have lifted and become firmer. Lower cheeks have a natural curve (my face has always been round), and the marionette lines have gone completely. There's zero sagging on my neck.

Age 58
After 13 years

September 2019

Exercise Schedule: 9 exercises 2 to 4 times per week.
I have a few more lines thanks to skin changes after menopause, but no deep wrinkles: the condition of my skin is fabulous. The brows are lifted, eyes are bright and open. My nose is neat, the cheeks are even more contoured and look slimmer. My face is firm and even though the jawline and neck take more work now, I still look younger than I did at 45!

Make-up this page. Left photo: Bourjois CC Cream, Shade 32, Blusher: unknown, Clinique Eyeliner: Charcoal, Max Factor Masterpiece Max Mascara, Lip gloss brand unknown.

Right photo: Bourjois CC cream, Shade 32, Clinique Powder: 20 Invisible Blend, RMS lip2cheek Blush: in Smile, Clinique Eyeliner: Black/Brown, Max Factor Masterpiece Max Mascara. Clinique Lip gloss: Adore U.

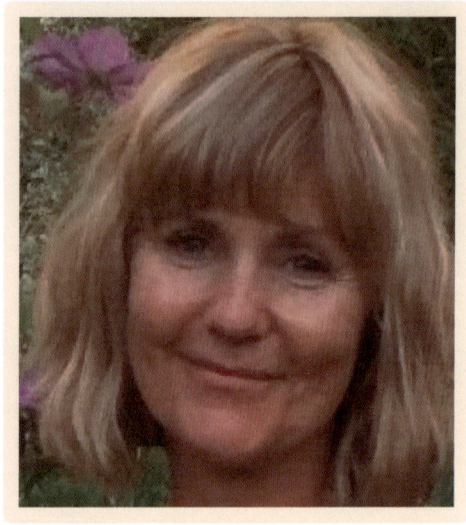 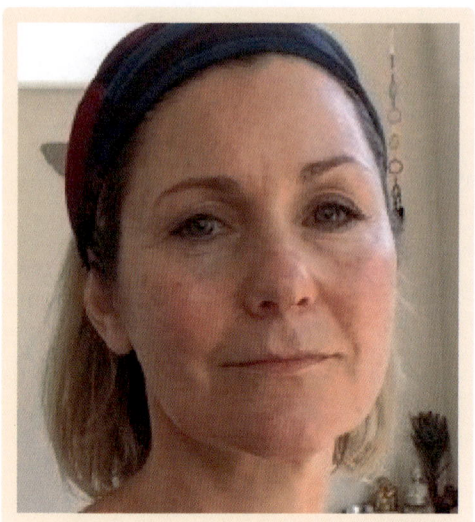

Dawn, UK

__Before: Left photo__. Taken a few years ago and although I have always practised yoga, I had never used Faceworks or any facial exercises before.

__After: Right photo__. Taken after my facial workout. I have no makeup on and have been doing Faceworks for around 12 weeks, usually 5x per week, I'm 48 years old. It doesn't really show in the picture but my lips are fuller (they used to be very thin) and the skin on my neck has tightened. My skin is clearer and I'm now looking for a lighter foundation with less cover. My cheeks have lifted and my frown lines on my forehead have diminished. I still have a few wrinkle issues around my eyes but I'm working on those! I am delighted with the Faceworks programme, and amazed at how effective these exercises are.

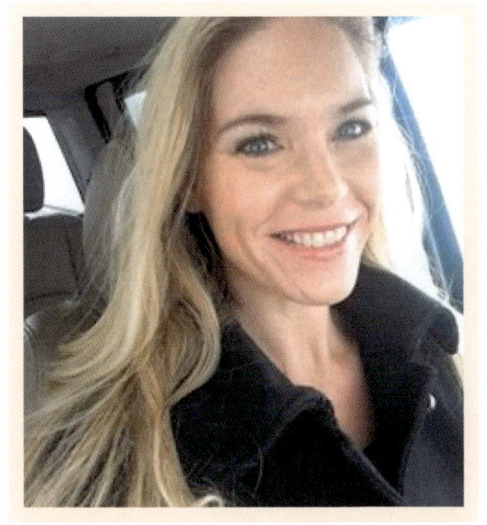 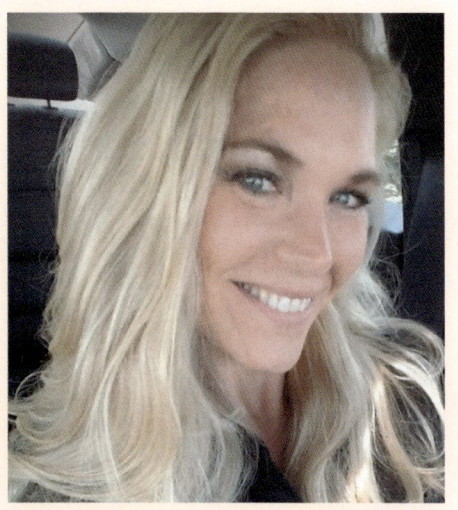

Kristine, USA

Before: Left photo. January 2016, before I started the exercises.

After: Right photo. I'm cancelling my appointment with the plastic surgeon: I don't need him anymore! I just finished week 9 and I'm absolutely loving my results! I love doing the exercises 'cause I know it's making huge changes to my face every time I do them.

Update from Kristine: I will look forever young because of Faceworks, I'm mistaken for 15 to 20 years younger than I am - I'll be 47 soon. I don't have wrinkles around my eyes or my forehead. My cheeks are lifted, my eye bags are gone and the muscles in my face are toned, lifted, strong. I feel the difference. Elaine, you deserve so much recognition for what you've created, I am forever grateful.

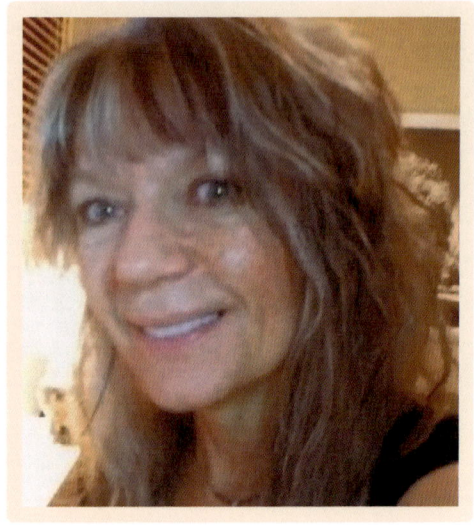
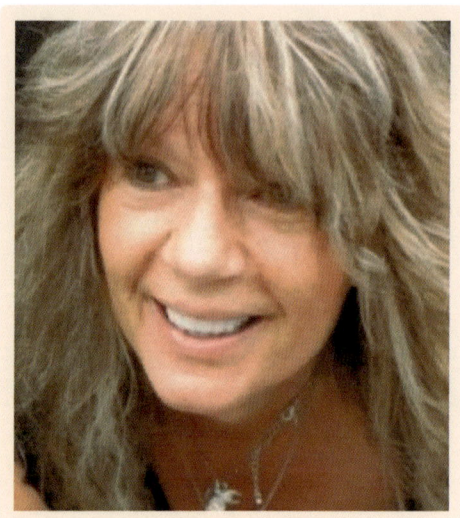

CharLee, Canada

Before: Left Photo. *I am thoroughly enjoying these exercises I am starting to see amazing results in the overall toning in my face, Thank you!*

After: Right Photo. *After doing your exercises for a year, I allowed my daughter to take a close up pic of me and was delighted with the results. I will be 59 years old May 7th and receive compliments daily. Thank You for having such an effective and enjoyable exercise routine & for keeping the muscles in my face toned and the woman in the mirror smiling back at me, Sincerely, CharLee*

There are a lot of people who have used the exercises for years, some since the program first went online in 2008. The age range is from mid-30s to around 90, and although the program is used mainly by women, there are a fair few guys too. Results for men are slightly different, and they report greater definition over the lower face and jawline.

More reviews are available on the website.

The Basics for Fabulous Faces

- **Skin Tightening**: The exercises work deeper than skin creams or serums. Circulation is boosted in deep skin layers, bringing blood and nutrients to improve the skin's condition. The result is firm, smooth skin, an even skin tone and a beautiful complexion.
- **Lines and Wrinkles**: Faceworks gives you a 'nip and tuck' without surgery by erasing folds and furrows. Existing lines and wrinkles are filled out, and the exercises help to slow down new signs of ageing from appearing by keeping the skin healthy.
- **Face Shape**: A neater, more youthful face shape emerges. Facial contours are defined and sculpted as the muscles rebuild and fill out loose skin. The correct balance of the face is restored to complement the features: lifted and toned over the cheeks and slimmer and tighter at the mouth and jawline.
- **Eyebrows:** Higher, arched brows and smoothed frown ridges open and frame the eyes for a fabulous new look.
- **Eyes**: the eye exercises target all the signs of ageing: deep crow's feet and wrinkles, sagging eyelids, dark circles, eye bags, under-eye hollows and puffy eyes.
- **Cheeks**: Quite simply, 'A List' cheekbones. The cheek exercises lift, sculpt and reshape for fabulous definition.
- **Lips**: Plumper, rosier lips without using fillers.
- **Jawline**: The exercises erase folds from nose to mouth, and reduce deep lines and loose skin. Sagging and jowls around the mouth are reduced, the jawline is defined and firm.
- **Chin**: Double chins and loose skin under the chin both improve for a slimmer, neater appearance

The exercises tone and restructure facial muscles by precise use. As the tissues under the skin become firmer, the skin visibly firms and lifts to improve facial contours. The transformation in appearance completely renews the face, but of course is entirely natural.

The 12 exercises in the Complete Workout will take 30 minutes or less to do, when you know them. Expect to take about 35-40 minutes while you're learning. If you're wondering if there are enough exercises in the Complete Workout to make a difference, the answer is yes, there are. They're designed to work the face thoroughly. The second book has more exercises for the lower face, plus advanced positions to give variety to your workout.

The Express Workout takes 6 exercises from the Complete Workout for a faster full face workout. Used singly, they also give an 'instant boost' for eyes, cheeks, lips or skin.

The Mini Workouts take 4 exercises from the Complete Workout to lift a single area of the face.

The 6 workouts take the guesswork out of which exercises to choose but if you'd prefer to make your own, use the Quick Lists. The program is designed to be versatile to suit what you need; whether that's a few exercises to enhance one place, or to give yourself a complete facelift.

So now you know the basic details of the program, we'll get on to what you want to know: how can Faceworks help *you*?

> *All of a sudden everyone is telling me how GREAT I look, my eyes look good, and I look younger! Thank you for your innovation in this whole area...if more people only knew what was available! I knew I would never brave the 'knife', and in reality it is always evident when one has had 'work', don't you think? But this is so natural; yet very effective...I could go on and on!"* Sally, USA

Part One

About You

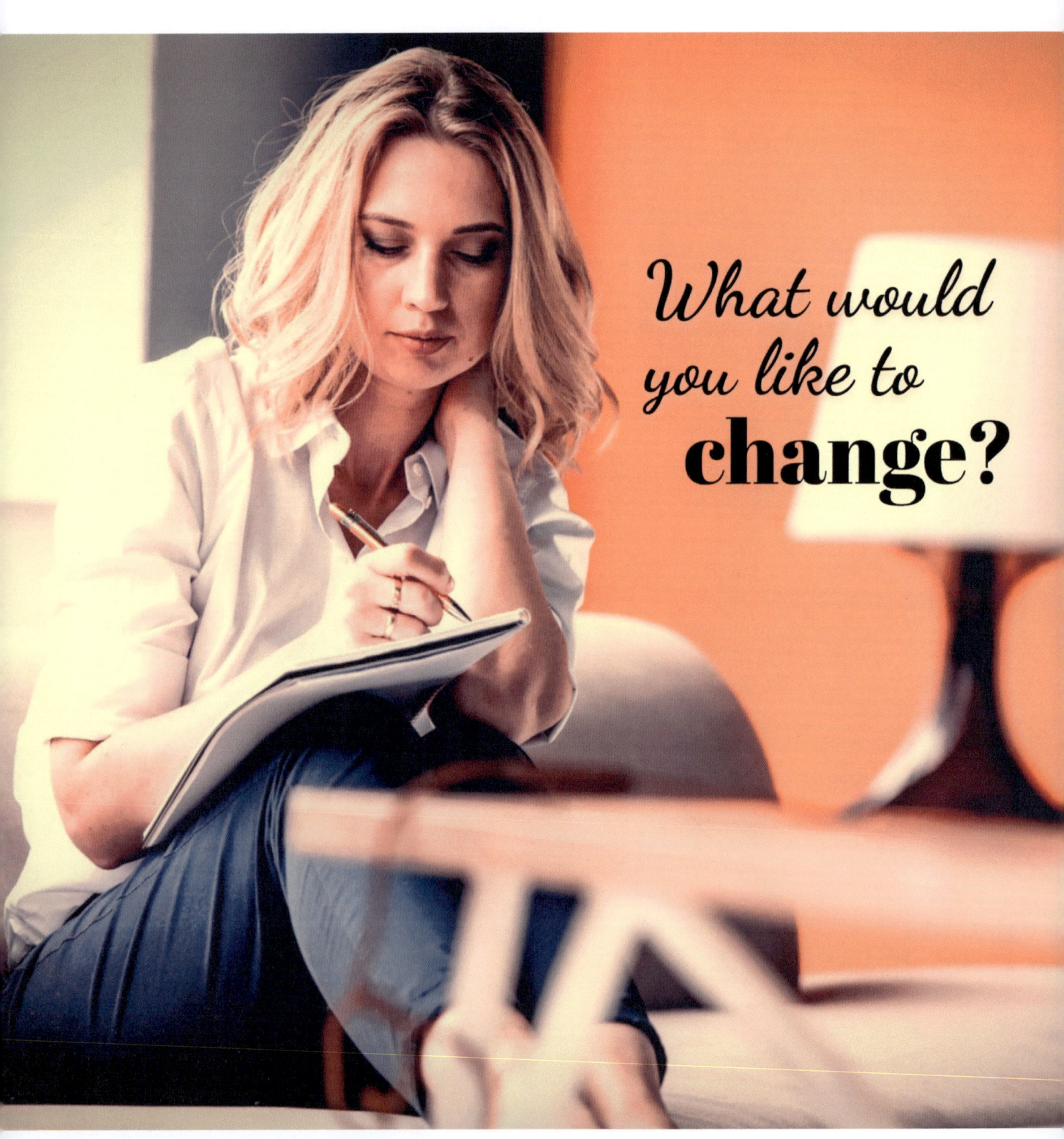

About You

What Would You Like to Change?

You may be very definite about the parts of your face you'd like to change, or you may just have a feeling of dismay when confronted by your reflection in the mirror. Either way, evaluating how you look right now will enable you to set a goal to work towards, allow you to monitor the changes and give you motivation.

Your Personal Reasons for Looking Better

Take a minute to really think about your personal reasons for wanting to change: be as honest as you can. Would you like to feel more confident or happier? Do you need a new look to begin a new phase in your life? You may have lost weight and feel your face needs a boost, to look fresh for a new job, or revamp yourself for some serious Va Va Voom. Another aspect to think about is how looking different might open up life in new ways: 'When I have my facelift, I'll feel/do/be able to…what? Search for that feeling of absolute, toe-tingling joy. When you have it, fix it in your mind. Write your toe-tingling reason(s) on post-it notes and stick them up where you'll see them. If you get too busy, too tired or just too plain lazy for Faceworks, they'll be powerful reminders.

Identify Your Goal

Is it your end goal to look great, or will looking great enable you to achieve your goal? 'Your personal reason' above might have already answered this for you, but if not take a moment to think about the motivation behind your need to look better. The more important the goal is to you, the higher your chance of success.

One lady; I'll call her Sue, who I used to see for Kinesiology sat down sadly after her treatment and said "I just want to look young and beautiful again". Her statement became my goal: it was the reason I started Faceworks. If ever I came up against a problem, I only had to remember how she looked as she said those words, and it was enough to make me press on. Needless to say, she had the program free of charge when it was finished.

Be precise about your goal, even if it's only that you want to get rid of your jowls by Christmas. If your goal is an event such as a wedding, don't forget the bonus of looking great after the event. See the wider picture to the time beyond, when the exercises keep your face looking toned and healthy. I'm presently 13 years on from achieving my goal and the confidence boost from looking great never fades.

It's no coincidence that on the Faceworks' website, the busiest month is January, with all the frantic reinventing that goes on in the New Year. If your decision and your goal are clear, then the doing is (almost!) effortless.

Do You Dare to Look Great?
A percentage of people who buy a workout from the website never start the program, it's almost as if they are too afraid to try. Whatever their reason for wanting to make changes, they don't believe in *themselves* enough to carry things through. It's like buying a fabulous outfit and never wearing it, or having a gift voucher for a beauty treatment and never getting around to booking at the salon.

Don't let 'Can'tbebothered-itis' run your life. Have the courage to look fabulous: why shouldn't you look downright sensational? Nobody gets prizes for being a shrinking violet. I'm reminded of this when I see people who seem to adore being noticed: who have the confidence to stand out and turn heads. Most people have the odd day when they feel like this. Being in control of ageing and knowing you look good can have a profound effect on other aspects of your life, too. Remember it's within your reach to feel fabulous *every* day.

Sometimes it isn't the fear of failure that stops us achieving, it's the fear of success. Change is good, and change because of looking great is even better! If you put the work in and follow the program, change will come. It's nothing to be frightened of.

> *"You've really changed my life! I've noticed such a positive improvement with the exercises. A thousand thanks."* Coco

Find Your Face Shape

If you're over 40, it's likely that the shape of your face will have altered since you were in your 20s and this review should prove helpful. Oval and triangular face shapes are often where most of us start out when we're younger and the final two types are the shapes that tend to develop as we get older, after facial sagging develops. You'll use your face shape in the next step.

Take your hair away from your face with a hairband or hairclip – you want to be able to see the outline of your whole face without any hair in the way. Don't smile because this alters the shape. Study your face and see which of the following you match most closely:

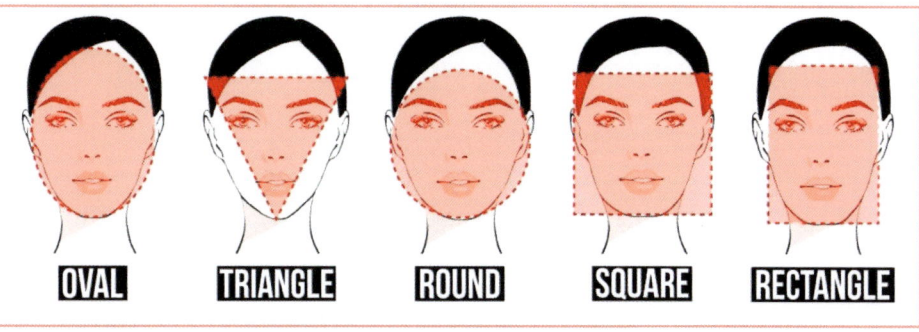

Oval: the length from top to bottom is greater than the widest point across the cheeks. The jaw and forehead are rounded, the sides are gently curved.

Triangle: the widest point of the face is across the forehead, the chin is the narrowest part of the face.

Round: the width across the cheekbones is around the same as the length of the face and the outline is full or curved with no sharp angles.

Square: the forehead and jaw are the same width, and the length of the face is roughly the same as the width. This face shape has more sharp angles than a round face.

Rectangle: the face is longer than it is wide. The width is the same across both cheekbones and chin. The sides are straight, and the jawline is roughly square.

How You Look Now

Without being overly critical study your face in a mirror in natural daylight. Artificial light or bright sunshine casts shadows and doesn't give a true representation.

Fill in the 'How you look now' list opposite using the notes below as a guide:

1. Eyebrows: are your brows arched, flat, drooping, or too low? Is the space between them lined or ridged?
2. Eyes: do they look tired: is the top eyelid covered by the skin under the brow? Are there any folds on the outer edge, deep lines or crows' feet? What do the lashes look like?
3. Under Eyes: note down if you have shadows, hollows, eye bags, loose skin, deep lines, etc.
4. Cheeks: too thin and flat, too full and rounded? Is the skin heavy, loose, or sagging?
5. Lower Cheeks: is this area too heavy, plump, gaunt or just shapeless?
6. Mouth: thin lips, or lips without shape? Are there deep expression lines, or folds that run from the corners of your nose down to the corners of your mouth?
7. Chin: note down if you have a double chin, 'marionette' lines from the corners of the mouth to the chin.
8. Jawline: is there too much 'weight' here as your face has dropped over time, or is the jawline undefined?
9. Skin: note down any skin problems such as dryness or breakouts and patchy skin tone. What is the texture like: dry, papery, uneven, etc? Is the colour good, pale, sallow or tired-looking?
10. Face Shape: oval, triangle, round, square or rectangle? Is it different to how it used to be?

Although you might feel despondent about some of the things you've written down, don't worry. This is your starting point. Now you know what you have to work with, take a deep breath and let it go, the hard part is done: it's time to move on to your Wish List.

How you look now

- EYEBROWS
- EYES
- UNDER EYES
- CHEEKS
- LOWER CHEEKS
- MOUTH
- CHIN
- JAWLINE
- SKIN
- FACE SHAPE

Your Wish List

This time you're going to decide what you want to achieve. If you're over 40, use a photo from 10 years ago. Results from the exercises can be dramatic but they will follow the natural structure of **your** lovely face, not someone else's. So if you have dreams of (insert celebrity name)'s doe eyes, tiny nose, etc. remember Faceworks is good, but only surgery can alter your bone structure.

Once again, study your face; then fill in the 'Wish List' using the points below as a guide:

1. Eyebrows: what kind of shape do you want; a higher arch; just generally lift, a better shape? Do frown lines or furrows need to go as well?
2. Eyes: what needs improving on the top lid, what changes do you want on the outer corner? Would you like brighter, more open eyes, lifted lids, less sagging, curvier lashes?
3. Under eyes: how would you like this area to look: reduced hollows or bags? Do you want to plump the area and add volume, smooth the skin, firm and tone as well?
4. Cheeks: higher, a slimmer look, more sculpted, increased volume, not so flat and saggy, toned, tighter skin?
5. Lower Cheeks: write down if you'd like this area to look neater, slimmer, more toned, perhaps reduce the heaviness and sagging.
6. Mouth: plumper lips, more shape, erase folds and deep expression lines; reduce vertical lines in the top and/or bottom lips.
7. Chin: do you want to firm this area, reduce jowls or a double chin, plus maybe reduce folds or deep lines?
8. Jawline: improve the line of the jaw, reduce loose skin or define the jaw?
9. Skin: would you like to improve how skin looks, increase firmness, smoothness, reduce dryness, plus have skin that looks healthier?
10. Face Shape: do you want to slim or tone up the overall shape, or go back to the face shape you had when you were younger?

Tip: Photos are a good way to monitor your progress. Take one before you start the program, and at the end of your first, second and third month. Use the same location and light each time.

Transferring your 3 dimensional face to a 2 dimensional image often results in a loss of fine detail, so don't be surprised if the photos don't show all the changes that are physically there in real life.

Your wish list

- **EYEBROWS**
- **EYES**
- **UNDER EYES**
- **CHEEKS**
- **LOWER CHEEKS**
- **MOUTH**
- **CHIN**
- **JAWLINE**
- **SKIN**
- **FACE SHAPE**

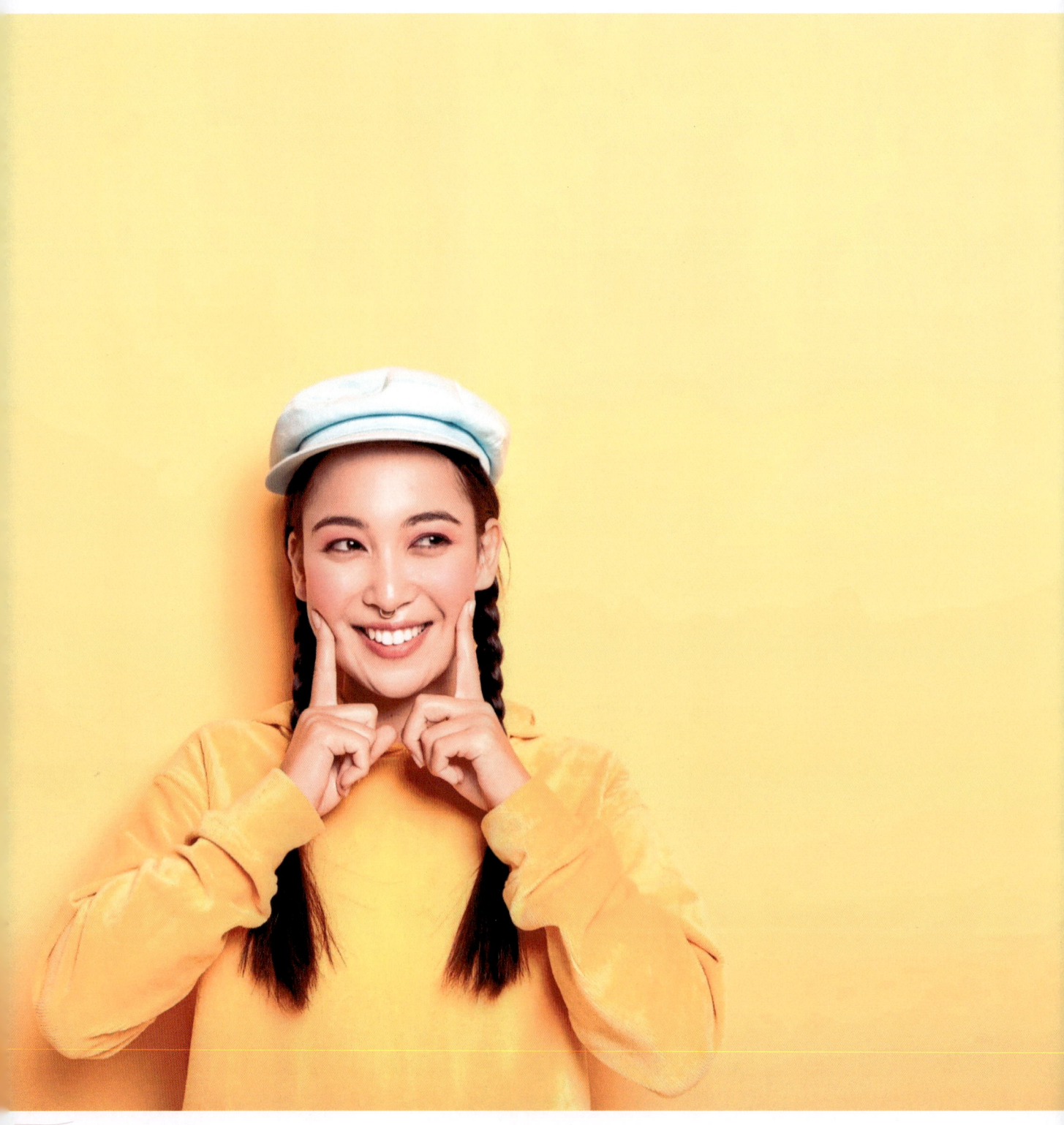

Part Two

The Face Exercises

As with any new exercise program, it is advisable that you check with your GP to make sure the Faceworks exercises are suitable for you, even if you consider yourself to be fully fit. If you have any past or current injuries, or any medical condition that requires professional care or medication, please be safe and seek advice before beginning the program.

As the program also includes eye exercises, it is also advisable that you check with your optician for similar reasons.

Workout Videos

All these exercises are on video at: www.faceexerciseguru.com. The website has all 6 workouts listed in this book, and all come complete with an easy to follow course.

The Face Exercises

How to Get Your Facelift

By now you have probably flicked through the first pages, looked at the exercises, tried some of them and used the Quick Lists to find the ones you need for your least favourite places. And perhaps there's a thought about how many exercises you can get away with *not* doing, so you don't use up too much of your time.

It is the repetitive nature of exercise that causes change to happen. It would be great if one sit-up a day was enough to develop a six-pack, but muscles only tone up with regular use. To change how you're ageing, you have to change what you're doing.

The 12 exercises in the Complete Workout give a complete facelift; together they work all facial muscles comprehensively. The Express Workout is a shorter full face workout, and if you only have one place you'd like to change, use a Mini Workout. Or mix and match the exercises to suit what you'd like to achieve: maybe eyes and a little bit of skin boosting, for example, or lips and brows, etc. Use the program to get the results you'd like: even one exercise done regularly will give you results.

If you're over 45 it's very likely that you'll see the best results with the Complete Workout. This is because, no matter how good your skin care regime, muscles will be starting to sag. Some of our trial participants were in their mid-30s, so ageing happens sooner than you might think.

The following pages assume that you'll be using all of the exercises, so mentally amend where necessary to suit your choice of workout.

> *"I started doing your exercises a week ago and already my nose and eye area feel less 'bony' and plumper...so nice! I am 63 years old and for the past 5 years have felt so frustrated about my facial sagging and had no idea how to change it." Louise, USA*

Kick Start Your Facelift

However you decide to use Faceworks, there's one thing you need to get those results coming: dedication. Set a date in your diary, phone, etc. for three months' time and commit to doing your workout 5 times a week, every week for those 12 weeks.

If you can't commit the time right now, wait until you can. The first three months are crucial: you really do need those 5 workouts every week. The muscles have to be worked regularly and consistently so that they change their shape and lift, and that won't happen if you stop and start or only work out a few days here and there.

All of the workouts have the same schedule of one workout on 5 days every week.

After the first intensive phase: those very special 12 weeks, you can reduce the workout schedule to between 3 to 4 times a week. The muscles will still be worked enough for them to improve in condition, though the lifting and toning will continue at a slower pace. Faceworks is designed to fit your needs. The program can be stepped up or down as you like; step it up to look your stunning best for those times when it really matters, reduce it to 3 to 4 times a week to maintain your facelift.

> *"I am astounded! I have exercised my face for several years using several programs, and I have NEVER seen such quick results. In only a couple of days, the corners of my mouth are level, after staying downturned through years of facial exercise. I am so thrilled with my lips."* Cathy, USA

How to Space Your Workouts

Muscle fibres rebuild after exercise and it is best to have a regular schedule so your facial muscles get time to rest and recuperate. The 5 times a week program gives you two rest days to be taken when you like: both together or one day at a time.

The program is safe to do every day, though please ease in slowly if you want to do this. Start with 5 times a week for the first month, then add one extra day at a time to allow the muscles to strengthen and get used to doing more.

Tip: make your Faceworks 'me' time with a little peace and quiet. Resist checking your phone or feeding the dog, and relax while you exercise.

Fit Faceworks into a Busy Life

Make Faceworks work for you and it won't be just another chore to get done. For example, take advantage of the circulation boosting effect to wipe away tiredness first thing in the morning, or to ease tension and relax you in the evening. If you're going out, use your exercise session as a home facial before you go out, and wait for the compliments to start rolling in.

I've used my workouts while writing this book to get my brain working and clear my thoughts, and it has worked exceptionally well. Usually, I use a regular time before I start work. Whenever you decide to make space in your day, make it a cast-in-stone habit.

Keep Your Facelift for Life

When you are happy with how you look, maintaining your facelift takes less time. With each exercise taking no more than a couple of minutes, it gives the ability to fit even a whole set of 12 exercises into those gaps in your day when you have 5 or 10 minutes to kill. Notice I said 'gaps'- exercising while doing something else cuts concentration down and you'll find yourself making faces without achieving anything. The muscles need your full attention, not half or even three-quarters: I've tried to multitask with the exercises and it doesn't work, so give yourself the luxury of a break and your face will thank you for it.

Probably the most unusual query I've had was from someone who wasn't getting very good results – it turned out she did her exercises on a busy train into work every day while squeezed in between other commuters.

Remember: solitude and quiet = concentration = results.

Tip: Refresh your workout every 6 months and go back to basics. Muscles get lazy! Get a mirror and go through the workout as if you're beginning again. Even I do this and without fail, realise I'm doing things wrong or muscles have stopped pushing as hard as they should.

> *"I have been doing Faceworks for four months, and the results are amazing. My brows have lifted, my lips are plumper, my jowls and naso-labial folds are so much better, my cheeks are high and round again, and I have amazing cheekbones. I am 48 going on 49, and Faceworks has transformed and rejuvenated my sad, slightly sagging face, so I now look fresh and full of energy. For the first time in years I can look in the mirror and be happy with what I see, and that is a miracle as I see it." Jette, Denmark*

Faceworks Diary

The following Faceworks Diary pages are for you to fill in at the end of each week, from Week 1 to Week 12 of the program.

When you've filled in the results at end of week 5 or 6 in the Diary, check back to the Wish List to see how far you've come. Do the same at the end of week 8 or 9 and tick the points on the Wish List you've achieved. Usually (but not always), the upper part of the face lifts fastest and will be closer to your Wish List than the middle and lower face. Use the same kind of light to compare each time, so that you get a true comparison to see how your facelift is progressing.

Repeat the comparison at the end of week 11 or 12. By this time, the middle and lower face should have caught up with the top. Results may be slower if you're 50+: the Results Timeline (after the Diary pages) has more on this.

The Results Timeline will help you to see what you can expect and if you're on track with your facelift and moving away from where you began on the 'How you look now' list. If you are not seeing the improvements you think you should, review the How to do Faceworks and the Solutions for Problems sections. Seeing the exercises in real time on video on the website is another option.

If you achieve all the points on the Wish List before 12 weeks, move onto the maintenance schedule outlined at the end of the Results Timeline under 'Three Months Plus'.

When we carried out our client trial, each person had the Diary to fill in. Seeing the progress in black and white was surprisingly exciting for everyone, myself included. Another plus was that writing the progress down helped the trial participants to keep up with their schedule, and gave them a record of the improvements throughout the 12 weeks. If the trial was anything to go by; it should give you a welcome feeling of achievement as you work towards your goal. The age group for the trial was from mid 30s to 50 years, and all participants saw noticeable changes.

If you receive a comment about how you look, write that down too. Often it is the people who don't see you every day who notice that something about you has changed.

Tip: Ask a friend or family member to help monitor your progress. Choose someone who you can count on to give you an honest answer, and who is generally observant. It's best if they don't see you too often: once a week or every 2 weeks is about right.

Faceworks Diary

Cross off the days you do Faceworks on the M T W T F S S strip. Fill in the results in the boxes. For example, at the end of week 1, note down the changes for your brows and eyes next to 'Brows & Eyes' under 'Week 1'. Continue to record your results every week, even if it's simply 'less tired' or 'healthier' & *definitely* if someone's tells you that you look well.

Cross days off →	**WEEK 1** M T W T F S S	**WEEK 2** M T W T F S S	**WEEK 3** M T W T F S S
EYEBROWS & EYES	*write results here*		
UNDER EYES & CHEEKS			
LOWER CHEEK & MOUTH			
CHIN & JAWLINE			
SKIN & FACE SHAPE			

Faceworks Diary

Cross off the days you do Faceworks on the M T W T F S S strip. Fill in the changes in the boxes. Use the Results Timeline to check for the results you should see. On Week 5 or 6, check back to your Wish List to see how far you've come.
Tip: ask a friend to help you monitor changes every week or two weeks - a fresh pair of eyes is useful.

	WEEK 4 M T W T F S S	**WEEK 5** M T W T F S S	**WEEK 6** M T W T F S S
EYEBROWS & EYES			
UNDER EYES & CHEEKS			
LOWER CHEEK & MOUTH			
CHIN & JAWLINE			
SKIN & FACE SHAPE			

Faceworks Diary

Cross off the days you do Faceworks on the M T W T F S S strip.
Fill in the changes in the boxes.
Compare your results with the Wish List at Week 8 or 9 and mark the wishes you've achieved.

	WEEK 7 M T W T F S S	**WEEK 8** M T W T F S S	**WEEK 9** M T W T F S S
EYEBROWS & EYES			
UNDER EYES & CHEEKS			
LOWER CHEEK & MOUTH			
CHIN & JAWLINE			
SKIN & FACE SHAPE			

Faceworks Diary

Cross off the days you do Faceworks on the M T W T F S S strip.
Fill in the changes in the boxes. Week 12 is the end of the 'intensive' phase.
Compare your results with the Wish List on Week 11 or 12 and mark the wishes achieved.

	WEEK 10 M T W T F S S	**WEEK 11** M T W T F S S	**WEEK 12** M T W T F S S
EYEBROWS & EYES			
UNDER EYES & CHEEKS			
LOWER CHEEK & MOUTH			
CHIN & JAWLINE			
SKIN & FACE SHAPE			

Notes

Results Timeline

If you've done any kind of body exercise you'll know you often have to wait for a month or more to even begin to see the results of your hard work. You'll begin to see changes a lot faster for the face. The first effects of Faceworks are noticeable in around 6 to 10 days, with blooming skin and sparkling eyes at the top of the list. The full list of the changes you can expect and when is below.

We've had many people tell us their friends and colleagues have commented on how well they're looking after beginning the program – those early changes are not just wishful thinking! It gives such a confidence boost when your face starts to change. By two months you will look noticeably and still very naturally different, and be well on the way to your own facelift.

All the results have been collected from the research carried out during development of the program and from the client trial. The emails from people over the years echo this same journey through.

If you do all 12 exercises 5 times every week for 12 weeks, these are the changes you can expect to see – obviously if you're using the Express Workout, a Mini Workout or your own, the changes will apply to the places that are exercised.

Two Weeks

The overall appearance of the skin is the first response to exercise – the complexion starts to bloom; eyes are brighter and more open, skin problems less noticeable. Cheeks look subtly toned, lips are plumper and rosier and double chins less prominent. You'll look like you've had a really good night's sleep.

One Month

From the top of the face: eyebrows are higher with a noticeable arch and the skin between a little smoother; there is less droop on the top eyelids and on the outer corners, where the skin is lifting. Eyes are bright and open, the lash line appears enhanced, shadows and puffiness are reduced. The cheek muscles sit higher, and the front of the face is more contoured, with a hint of the shape to come. Lips are plumped with an enhanced upper lip shape and cupids' bow. Benefits to the skin have increased: the complexion is smooth, glowing and feels firmer to the touch. Lines and wrinkles are beginning to fill out. Skin problems like dryness and blemishes can be seen to be improving. Overall, there are definite but still subtle changes – your friends will ask you if you've been away or had a facial.

Two Months

Frown furrows are almost gone, hooded eyes and crow's feet are lifted and reduced. The eyes retain their brightness even if you're feeling tired. Under eye skin is toned and smoother with a reduction in bags and shadows. Hollows under the eyes are filled out, smoothing crepiness and lines. The cheek muscles have lifted to their true position, giving beautiful contours to the front and sides of the face. The balance of the face is noticeably different: higher and more youthful. Around the mouth, folds and deep lines are reduced by 40%; the lips are plump and rosy. Jawline and jowls are neater and will continue to lift. Double chins are reduced; the skin under the chin is smoother and tighter. Skin continues to improve. Skin feels and looks a lot firmer and healthier than before.

> *"I'd like to thank you for this very positive group of exercises. I have been doing them for 2 months now and see a big improvement. I had used a VERY well-known programme prior to this but was not happy with it"* Isobel, Scotland

Three Months

The lower face now shows a marked improvement: it takes until now for the muscles here to lift. As we get older, the facial muscles relax and sag down, creating heaviness around the bottom of the cheeks, jawline and mouth. When the cheeks lift completely, the sagging that has been hiding your true face shape is lifted away. Folds around the mouth, jowls and jawline improve dramatically as the skin 'drapes' properly over firm muscles. The lower face looks slimmer and neater. Cheeks look toned and sculpted. Further up the face, eye hollows and bags show further improvements as the tissues tighten. Frown furrows should now be erased completely. There is progressive improvement in lines and wrinkles around the eyes.

This is the end of the Intensive 12 week Phase: you can safely drop the number of workouts to between three and four a week, depending on your needs.

Three Months Plus

Doing your workout three to four times a week will continue to refine your facelift, especially around the mouth, jowls, jawline and skin. Depending upon your age, it can take a little more than 3 months for the lower face to finish toning. If this is the case for you, it is safe to continue with the 5 times a week schedule until you reach the level you want.

A workout two to three times a week will keep the muscles toned and prevent your face from dropping. The exercises bring more benefits the longer you do it. I noted changes to my own face over a time period of two years, where the results slowed down but did not stop happening. After two years, it seemed I had reached 'peak toning'. I have completely lost the frail, faded look my face used to have at 45. My face looks toned, lifted, incredibly smooth and stronger – healthier.

Once you have your facelift, use the exercises to suit whatever you're doing. They are designed to be used as **you** need them. Do more workouts before a special event when you want to look your best, and a couple of times a week when you're busy. You can use the whole set of exercises, do only a few, or use the Express and Mini Workouts to switch things around. If life gets in the way, even two or three exercises done regularly will keep the muscles active until a longer workout is possible

Tip: Maintain your facelift with a workout 2 or 3 times a week, and choose one or two exercises to do every day for the places that need an extra boost.

The Complete Facelift Workout

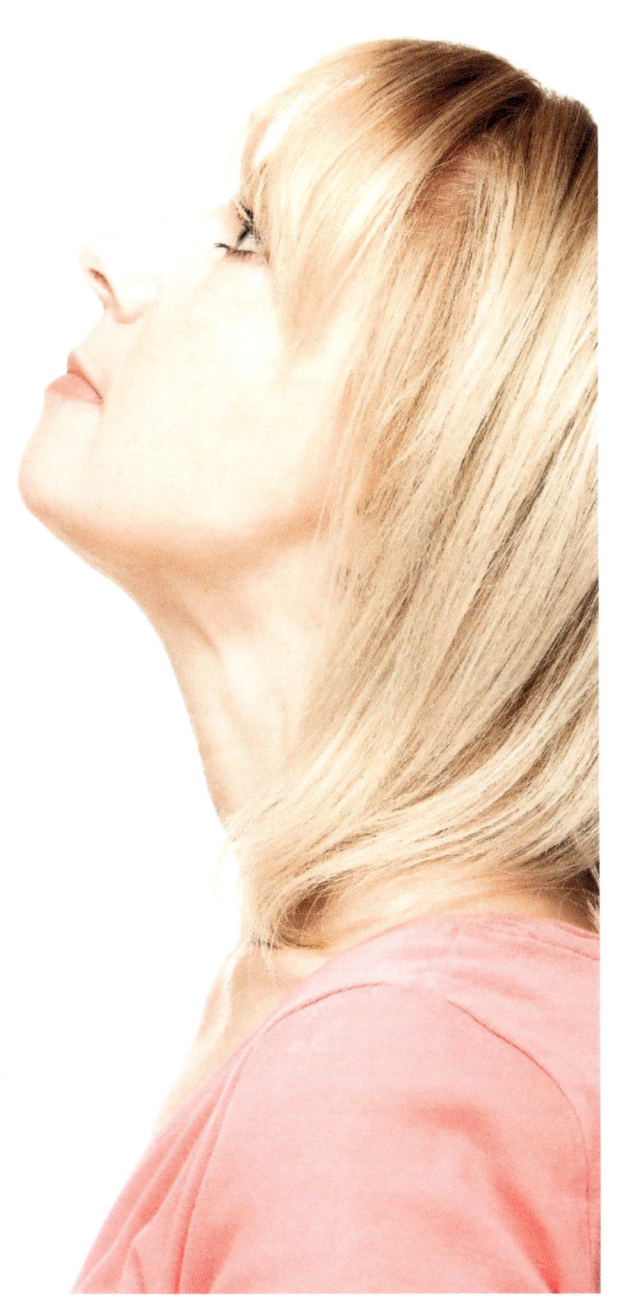

1. Facial Warm-up
2. Mouth Shaper One
3. Mouth Shaper Two
4. Lip Builder
5. Eyebrow Lift
6. Cheek Toner One
7. Eye Toner One
8. Eye Toner Two
9. Chin and Jaw Toner
10. Cheek Toner Two
11. Mouth Area Shaper
12. Face Finisher

How to do the Exercises

1.

Do the workout once a day. During the first 2 weeks, use a mirror every time as you learn the exercises, then twice a month after that to:

- Help you follow the exercises
- Check your positions are the same as in the photos.
- Make sure that the rest of your face is relaxed during each exercise.

Prop the book up next to the mirror so both are easy to see, the exercise instructions are in larger print to be easy to read. Don't be tempted to go over and over the exercises, after you've done the workout leave it until the next time. It will get easier as time goes on.

2.

Sit (or stand) to do the exercises with your shoulders relaxed and your back straight: perhaps do a couple of shoulder rolls backwards and forwards before you start. Good posture enables the neck vertebrae to move freely and makes the exercises easier to do.

3.

Each exercise isolates and targets specific muscles. Take your time, and carefully follow the instructions step by step. Check your position is the same as the photos at each step, before going on to the next. Learn slowly to get the foundations right, don't rush through.

4.

The Focus Point isolates and targets the right muscles, so you get the most out of each exercise. You don't need to worry about finding the right place because the Focus Point does it for you. The Focus Points are shown by a circle on the photos.

During Week 1, put a fingertip or two on the Focus Points (forget the finger positions on the eye and cheek exercises until Week 2 or 3). Using touch helps you feel the muscles contracting, and focuses your attention on the right place.

5.

Face muscles aren't used to working hard. To begin with, it might feel as though the muscles aren't doing anything at all: but don't worry. It takes 2 weeks or more for muscle fibres to build up enough strength feel a definite movement. As the fibres strengthen, the muscles contract more completely and are able to work harder. The workout becomes more effective, easier to do and takes less time.

6.

There's no need to make big, aggressive movements. Keep places other than the Focus Point relaxed: this takes a little bit of practice. Just remember no face scrunching! Screwing your face up prevents the muscles that *should* be working from doing what they need to. Face muscles are small: they need focused, precise movements to contract properly.

7.

After 3 weeks it's time to step it up a notch. When you hold the position, push the Focus Point muscles harder. Muscles are lazy: they will lift into the position for an exercise and just sit there unless your mind is engaged.

The real work to tone up the muscles is done **after** they are in position, they need to work hard once they're there. Keep the 'push' going at the Focus Point to the end of every repetition. Don't let the muscles slacken off at all, and check you're still doing the exercises without tensing up other parts of your face or your jaw.

8.

It's normal for your face to feel like it has been worked afterwards, and for skin to look plumped. A little muscle ache is expected. If your jaw feels tight, or if there's pain elsewhere, check the Problems (you'll find them after the Complete Workout). Any persistent pain shouldn't be ignored: stop exercising and see your doctor.

9.

Because 90% concentration is needed, don't multitask, believe me I've tried and it doesn't work! Despite that, Faceworks *is* designed to fit into your life. Be inventive with how you use your workout, and it won't be just another chore to get done. Some exercise time ideas:

- First thing in the morning
- As a beauty treatment before going out
- To relax you in the evening

It's best to do the whole workout from start to finish, but it can be split in two halves if there isn't time for one long session.

Exercise 1: Facial Warm-up

Focus Point: the cheek centres where the contraction is strongest: concentrate on pushing the muscles here

Good for: All neck and facial muscles, facial skin, and endocrine glands in the neck.

Time: 2.29 minutes

Benefits
This first exercise is based on the yoga 'Lion' asana. If you like; when you breathe out on point 2, visualise all stress and tension leaving your body with the out-breath.

This exercise warms the muscles in the face, lips, jaw and neck, in preparation for specific exercises. It improves the condition of the skin and stimulates blood and lymph flow to the larynx, trachea, thyroid and parathyroid glands. The deep breath stimulates the lungs and encourages relaxation.

This exercise repeats 5 times, as do the majority of the exercises in Faceworks. For each repetition of the exercise, hold the position at point number 6 for 15 seconds, or simply count silently and slowly to 10.

Do the exercises in front of a mirror so it's easy to copy the photographs.

Put your fingers on the Focus Points during the first week: shown by a circle on the photo.

Muscles Worked
All muscles from the cheekbones down to the base of the neck. Extending the tongue works the platysma at the front of the neck, and the deep jaw and neck muscles, including hyoid musculature under the tongue.

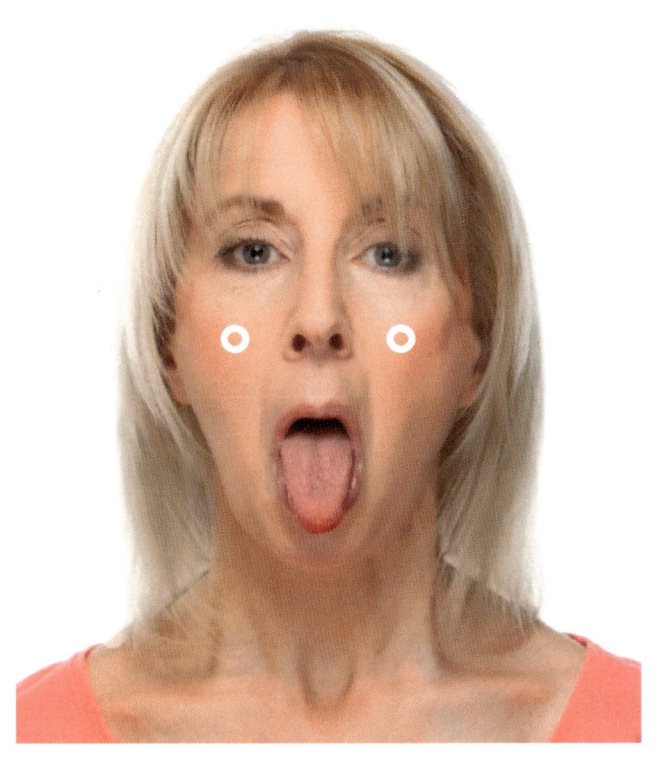

1. Sit straight and tall, with shoulders relaxed.

With the mouth closed, breathe in deeply through the nose.

2. Open the mouth into a long 'O' as you breathe out. Stretch the tongue out and point it down as far as feels comfortable.

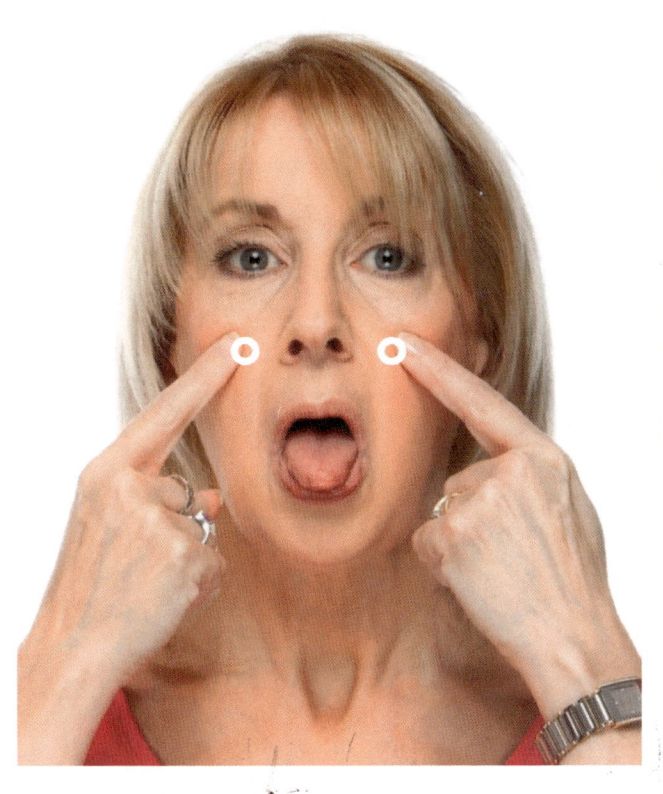

3. Place your fingers on the Focus Point as shown, to locate the muscles used next.

4. Contract your cheek muscles by lifting the corners of the mouth up: you should feel the cheeks tighten into little 'apples'.

5. Keep the mouth open and your tongue pointing down while you contract the cheeks for 15 seconds.

Relax and repeat 5 times.

Exercise 2: Mouth Shaper One

Focus Point: the mouth corners: keep pulling them up and out to maintain the stretch

Good for: Cheeks, naso-labial fold, lips, jowls, marionette lines, jawline and under the chin.

Time: 2.50 minutes

Benefits
The mouth is the first to benefit from this exercise: the lips shape up and mouth corners lift. Labial folds and grooves that run from the side of the nose to the mouth are reduced. Jowls, marionette lines and jawlines improve as the muscles under the chin and along the jawline are toned and tightened.

N.B. Do not clench the jaw, or roll the lower lip forward at all, keep a light pressure where the lips touch and save the effort to push the mouth corners up.

Muscles Worked
Orbicularis oris, risorius, zygomaticus minor and major, buccinator, masseter, platysma

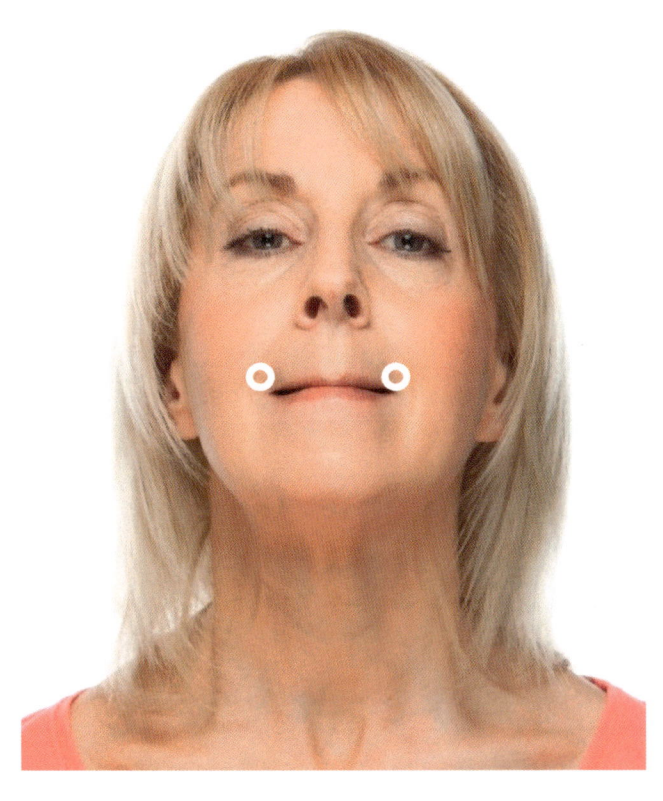

1. Roll the top and bottom lips over the teeth and close the mouth lightly, without pressure. Lift the chin slightly to make the exercise easier to do.

2. With the mouth still closed; pull the corners up into a wide smile as far as they will go. Don't worry if only the centre of your lips stay closed, it is normal to see gaps at the corners.

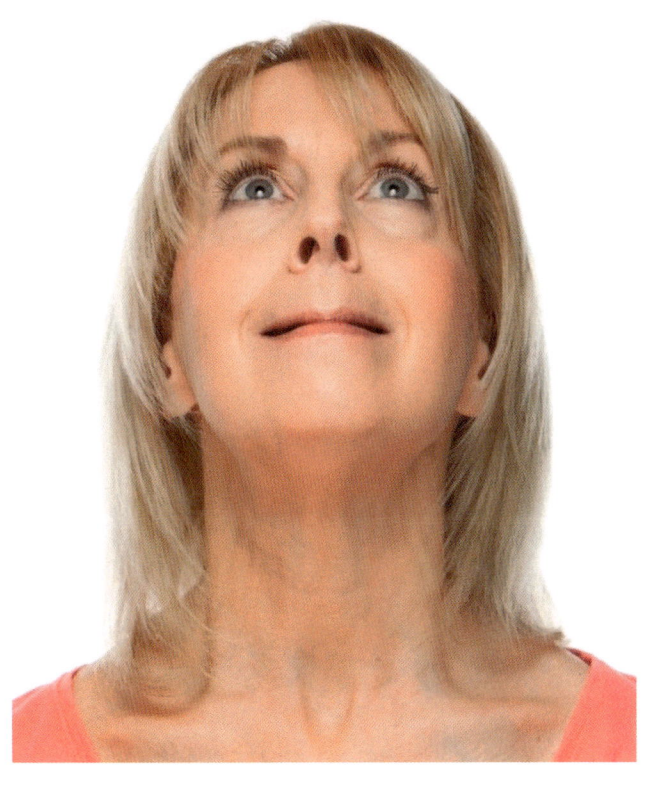

3. Keep lifting the mouth corners up. Don't allow the muscles to relax at all during the exercise.

4. The deep cheek muscles might ache, but there should not be any discomfort in the jaw joint. If there is, make sure you are only using the mouth corners to push up.

Hold for a slow count of 10, or 15 seconds.

Relax and repeat 5 times.

Exercise 3: Mouth Shaper Two

Focus Point: the area just above and below the lips, keep pulling the lips in to work the muscles properly

Good for: Vertical lip lines, expression lines around the mouth, folds and loose skin around the mouth.

Time: 2.35 minutes

Benefits
This exercise plumps lips beautifully and lifts the profile of the top lip, enhancing the cupids' bow. The plumping action fills out vertical lines in the top lip, and general expression lines around the mouth, tightening loose skin to erase folds. It improves circulation to the mouth and gives the nose tip a little workout too!

Muscles Worked
Orbicularis oris, zygomaticus major and minor, levator labii superioris, buccinator, platysma, depressor anguli oris, depressor labii inferioris, mentalis.

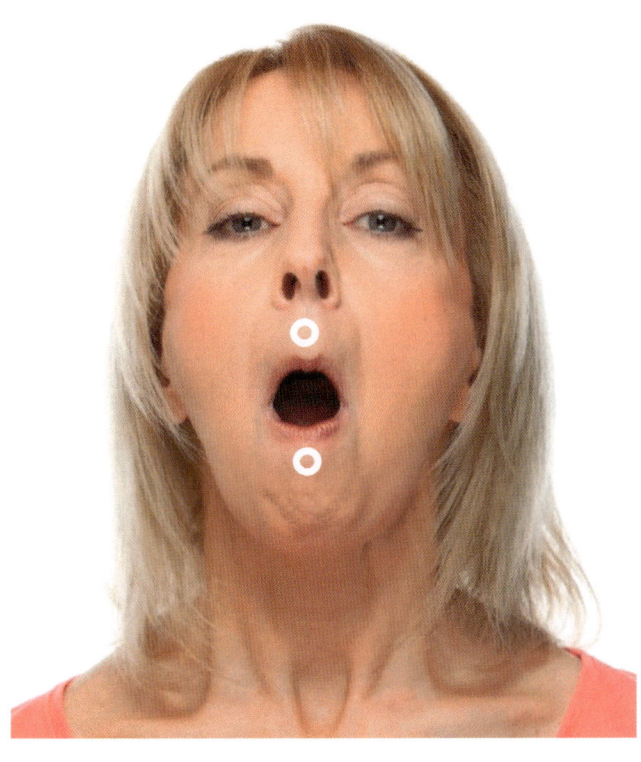

1. With your chin level, open your mouth into a long 'O'.

2. Roll both upper and lower lips over your teeth. Pull them in and round over your teeth until you feel the pull above and below the mouth.

3. Don't dig your teeth into your lips. Keep your mouth open in an 'O' and don't allow the pressure from your lips to close the mouth.

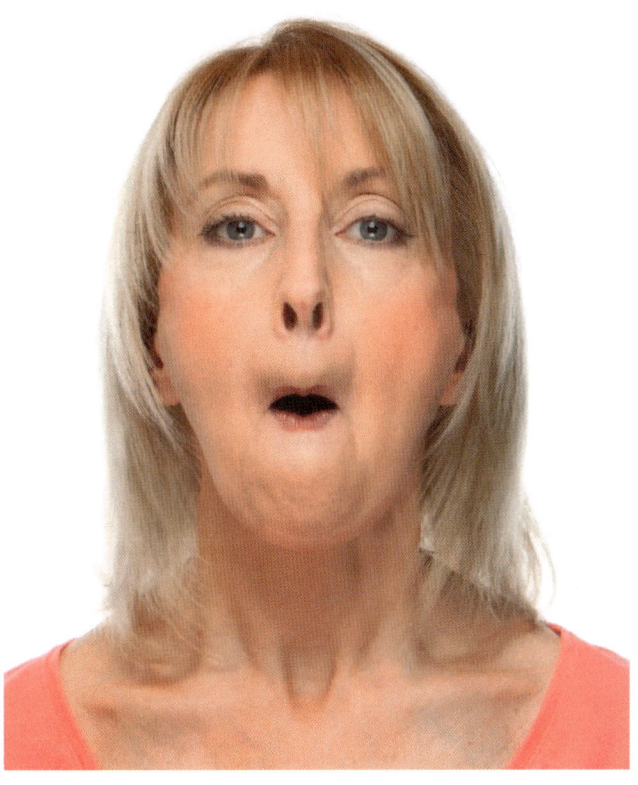

4. As you count slowly to 10, keep the lips trying to roll in all round the top, sides and bottom of the mouth. You will feel the muscles working even at the end of your nose, and on your chin.

Hold for a slow count of 10, or 15 seconds.

Relax and repeat 5 times.

Exercise 4: Lip Builder

Focus Point: the gap between your lips, leave the mouth open slightly to make the lip muscles work harder

Good for: defining the top lip line and cupids' bow and to give enhanced pout without fillers.

Time: 2.35 minutes

Benefits
The Lip Builder lifts and builds the top lip profile for a naturally enhanced pout. The bottom lip works hard and you should also feel the chin contracting. Finally, it tones the area around the sides of the nose. Lips are instantly plumped and 'rosier'.

If you have fine vertical lines on your top or bottom lip, see the tips over the page.

Muscles Worked
Orbicularis oris, buccinator, nasalis, zygomaticus major and minor, levator labii superioris, depressor labii inferioris, mentalis.

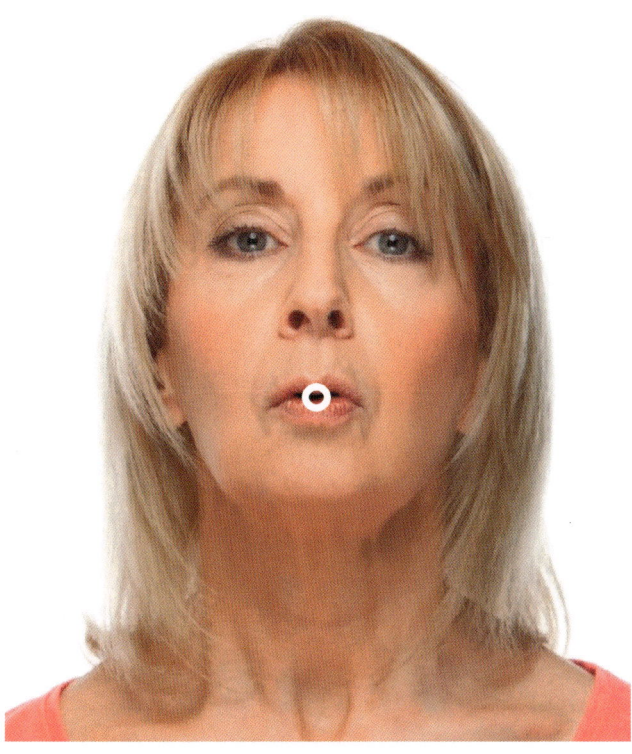

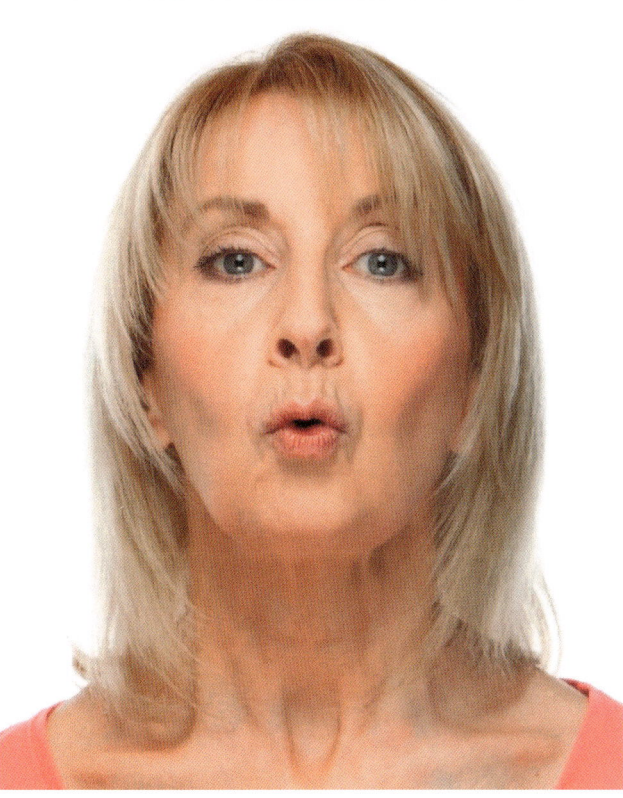

1. Sit straight with head level. Make a little pout with your lips, so there is a small gap between them.

2. Push both lips out, all the while concentrating on the little gap; until the lips are extended as far as they can go.

3. If it helps, put a fingertip between your lips to maintain the gap. Make sure the bottom lip is pushed out as far as the top one. Check the position in your mirror.

4. As you count to 10, keep your lips pushing out, as if you were trying to kiss someone on the other side of the room. See the next page if you notice vertical lines in your top lip.

Hold for a slow count of 10, or 15 seconds

Relax and repeat 5 times.

For existing lip lines:

If you have existing vertical lines in your top lip, or if they appear when you do the Lip Builder, either:

1. Use two fingers to smooth the lines out, as in the photo. It doesn't matter if you curl the lip out or apply a little pressure to the lip. If the muscles are still pushing out hard you won't stop them from working.

2. Or if your lips are capable, flare the top lip by curling it up.

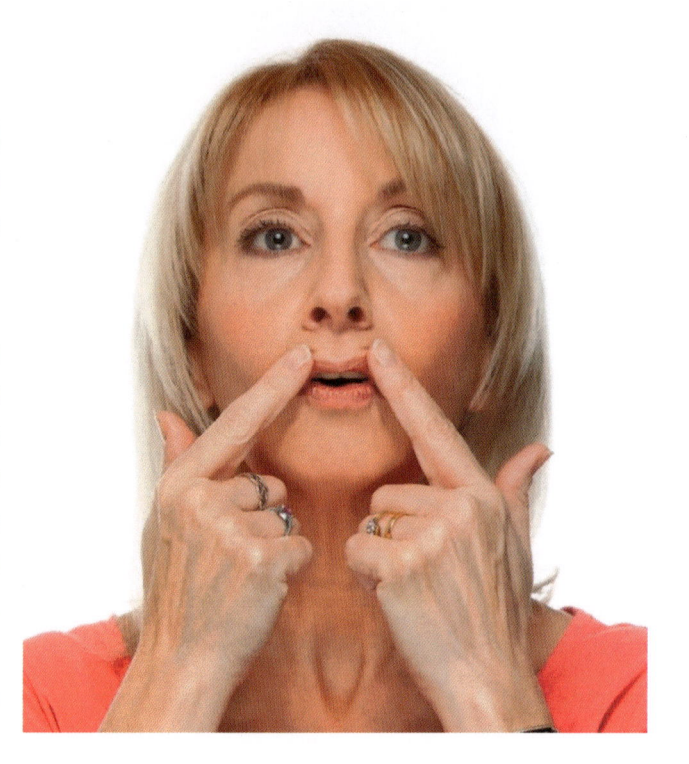

N.B. If neither of the above stop the lines, and they are still there as you push the lips out, leave this exercise out altogether and use Exercises 2, 3 and 11 to plump and shape the lips.

Exercise 5: Eyebrow Lift

Focus Point: Eyebrows- keep pushing them up and out, you'll find they will go up more than you would expect

Good for: drooping or flat brows, frown ridges and lines, hooded lids, tired looking eyes and crow's feet.

Time: 2.45 minutes

Benefits

Eyebrows to die for! High, defined and with a beautiful arch, the Eyebrow Lift reshapes the brows and erases frown ridges and furrows. As brows lift up; the space between the brow and eye increases, opening the entire eye area for dramatic results.

Muscles worked

Frontalis, galea aponeurotica, occipitalis, corrugator supercillii, procerus, posterior auricular.

1. Sit straight and tall with the chin level. Place one open palm lightly against the forehead just above the brows.

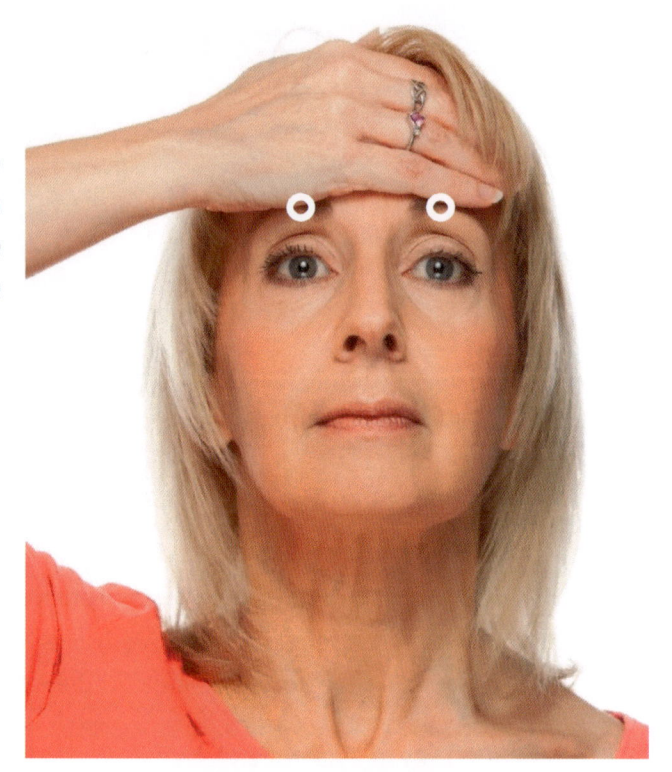

2. Raise your eyebrows up as far as possible, while gently lifting the flat palm against the skin to smooth out wrinkles on the forehead.

3. Do not push hard with your hand, the pressure is just enough to stop the lines from forming, and to isolate the brow muscles so they work properly.

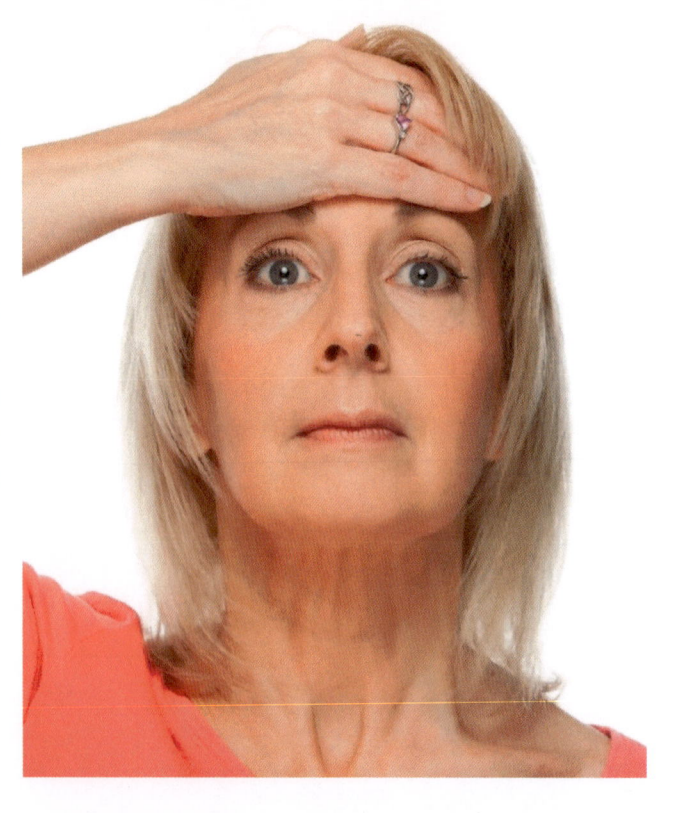

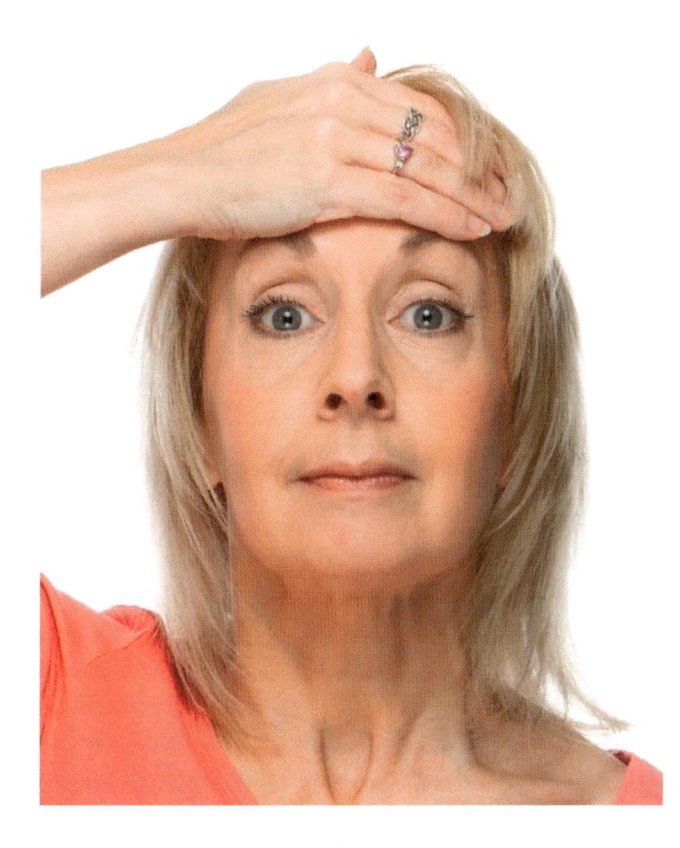

4. When the brows are up as far as you think they can go, keep lifting up and also **out** so the space between the brows gets a really good stretch. You might also feel the occipitalis muscle at the back of your head working too.

Keep lifting the brows for a slow count of 10, or 15 seconds.

Relax and repeat 5 times.

Leave the hand on your forehead if you prefer

If the lines on your forehead are in a different place, change the position of your palm, or use fingertips instead. We're all different physically, so adjust the position to suit you.

Exercise 6: Cheek Toner One

Focus Point: the middle and bottom of the cheek muscle. Push the muscles to work as hard as they can here

Good for: flat cheeks, heavy or chubby cheeks, loss of shape, loss of volume.

Time: 3 minutes

Benefits
Quite simply, this exercise gives you gorgeously contoured cheekbones even if you're not blessed with them naturally. It reshapes cheek muscles and lifts them up to sit **on** the cheekbone, instead of underneath it. This lift creates space under the cheekbone.

Sagging, flat cheeks are banished and cheek skin becomes firm and smooth. The weight of the face is gently altered to give a slim, neat lower cheek contour and new contours and definition to the front and sides of the face. This exercise is very effective for adding firmness and tone to chubby cheeks, and to correct loss of volume without using fillers.

Muscles Worked
Zygomaticus major and minor, levator labii superioris, risorius, buccinator.

Perfecting the movement
- Both the Cheek Toners use finger positions to ease out the skin - but if you're new to Faceworks, leave these out for the moment use your fingers to find the right muscles.
- Place your fingertips on the apple of your cheeks.
- Now open your mouth a little and then lift your top lip up into a smile - you should feel those muscles under your fingers bunch up a little. That bunching up is the muscles contracting to make your lips move.
- Practice doing this a few times, then when you can feel the muscles bunch up:
- Push your top lip up a little harder and hold the position for a slow count of 10. You'll find that the lip will naturally press on and slide up against the top teeth. Concentrate on the place in your cheeks where you feel the muscles working.
- Don't worry if your teeth show, and don't open your mouth all the way, otherwise the cheek muscles won't work as hard.
- Keep those eye muscles relaxed, use ONLY the cheek muscles to push the top lip up. Try not to screw your face up. If you notice your jaw feeling tight, relax it.
- At the count of 10, relax the muscles.

1. Sit with your back straight and chin level.

2. Place index fingers vertically alongside your eyes.

These finger placements are to *gently* smooth the skin around the eyes to prevent lines forming then the cheeks lift up.

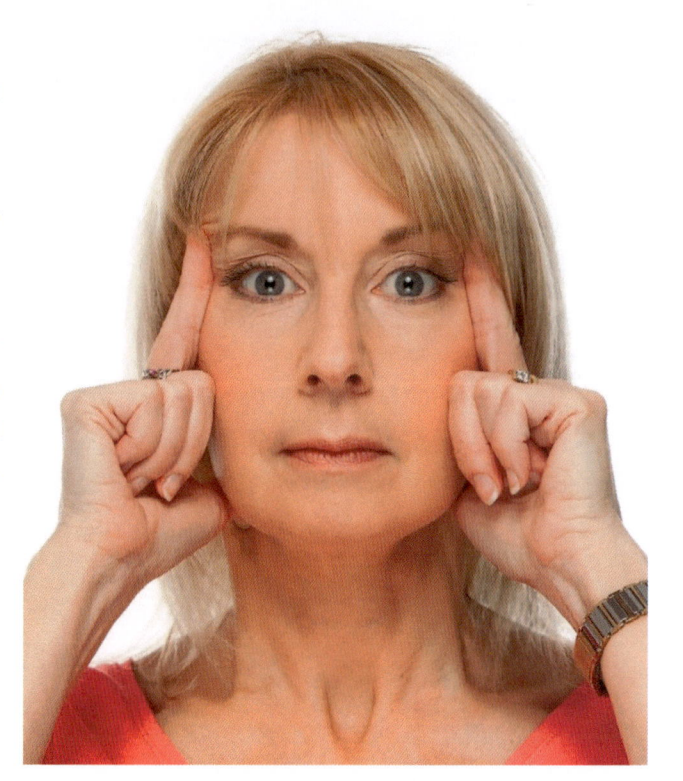

3. Place the middle fingers across, just under the lower lid.

In the first week, leave these finger positions out while you learn the exercise. Skip to point number 4.

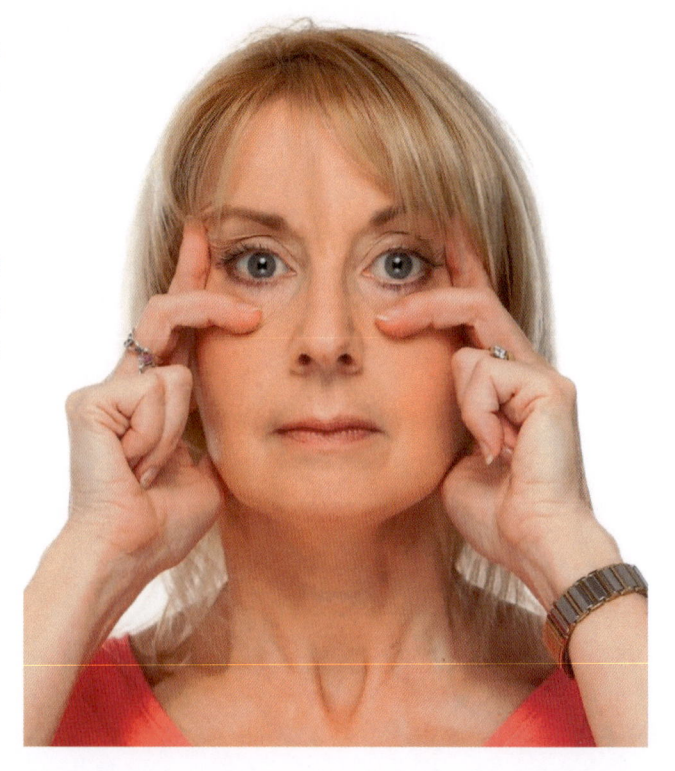

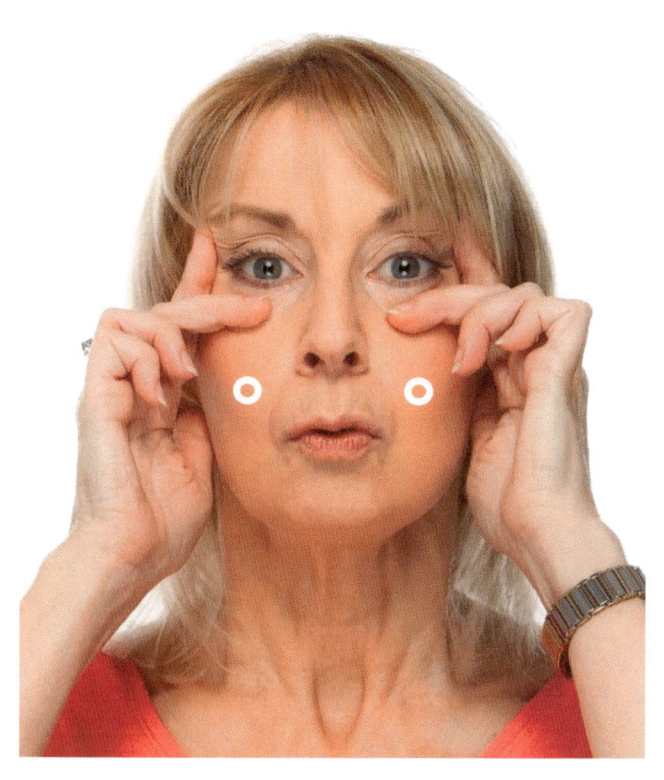

4. Now close your lips into a small pout with a gap in between, the same as in the Lip Builder (Exercise 4).

This moves the mouth into the right position to isolate the cheek muscles and lift them the right way.

The pout will disappear as you move the mouth in the next step.

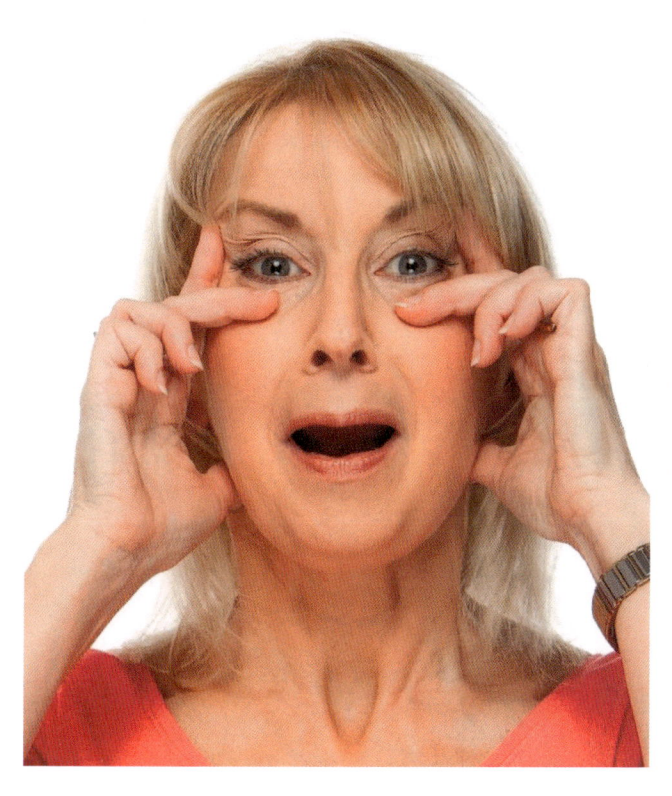

5. Now lift the top lip into a smile. You should feel and see the cheek muscles tighten and lift.

6. Drive the smile higher so the cheeks work hard.

7. Check your eyes and forehead aren't being used as well (they will try).

Hold for a slow count of 10, or 15 seconds.

Relax and repeat 5 times.

Creating Killer Cheekbones with the Cheek Toners

The cheek muscles are a large group of muscles, and rejuvenating them has a big impact on the overall shape of your face. When properly exercised, the change in cheek contours is noticeable from all angles. Until the age of around 30, cheek muscles sit on the cheekbone, but time makes them gradually slide lower. These exercises lift the muscles up and out to their original position, and the improved tone will give you high, toned cheeks and fabulous under cheekbone contours.

Slim and sculpt

Square and round faces often lack the 'sculpted' look that longer faces have, but with the Cheek Toners you can change that: they are brilliant at slimming down the sides and front of your face to get rid of the 'chubby' look so many people dislike. The widest point of any adult face should be across the top of the cheeks; not halfway down or lower. Cheek Toner One and Two will gently change the level of this widest point and raise it up to where it should be. As the muscles lift up and away from the middle of your face, the lower cheek area becomes slimmer and looks neater - more toned, and the entire shape of your face looks different.

Plump and volumise

Young faces have a cushioning layer of fat under the skin: it gives that fresh and dewy appearance and a natural curve to the cheek. It's a look many celebrities over a certain age try to achieve with fillers, but the results are often too extreme - and it has rightly earned the name of 'pillow face'. The Cheek Toners move the muscles up and out, but they do much more. With exercise, muscle fibres get tighter and plumper. Flat and sagging muscles literally rebuild and plump the skin naturally. These great exercises bring your natural curve back, without a filler in sight.

How can the Cheek Toners slim and add volume?

It's all to do with the position of the muscles. The slimming effect comes when the muscles lift: the 'up and out' movement slims down the face and takes the weight away from the lower cheek area.

The same lift increases volume in older faces that suffer from flat cheeks or hollows under the eyes. Both occur as cheek muscles lengthen and settle lower. It's the lack of padding at the top of the cheek that causes hollows, and often the lower ridge of the eye socket shows under the skin. When muscle fibres tone and lift back up; cheeks are restored to their original shape and condition, adding volume and structure.

Exercise 7: Eye Toner One

Focus Point: one inch under the eye at the top of the cheekbone

Good for: dull eyes, eye bags, hollows and shadows, lines and wrinkles, tired looking eyes, flat looking skin.

Time: 3 minutes

Benefits

This exercise rebuilds the under eye area and the lower lid. The lash line is defined; the eyes open up and begin to sparkle. Eye bags, hollows and shadows are all reduced and the skin becomes smoother as the tissues underneath firm and tone up. Lines and wrinkles are plumped out. Signs of tiredness that become etched around the eyes gradually fade, to reveal a brighter, younger, rejuvenated appearance.

When you begin Faceworks, only do 2 or 3 repetitions instead of 5 to avoid overworking the muscles (overworked eye muscles sometimes cause an eye strain type headache).

Muscles Worked

Orbicularis oculi, corrugator supercillii, levator palpebrae superioris.

1. You can either keep your chin level, or raise it slightly, whichever is easiest. Use the finger positions for Cheek Toner One for this exercise if you notice the skin wrinkling.

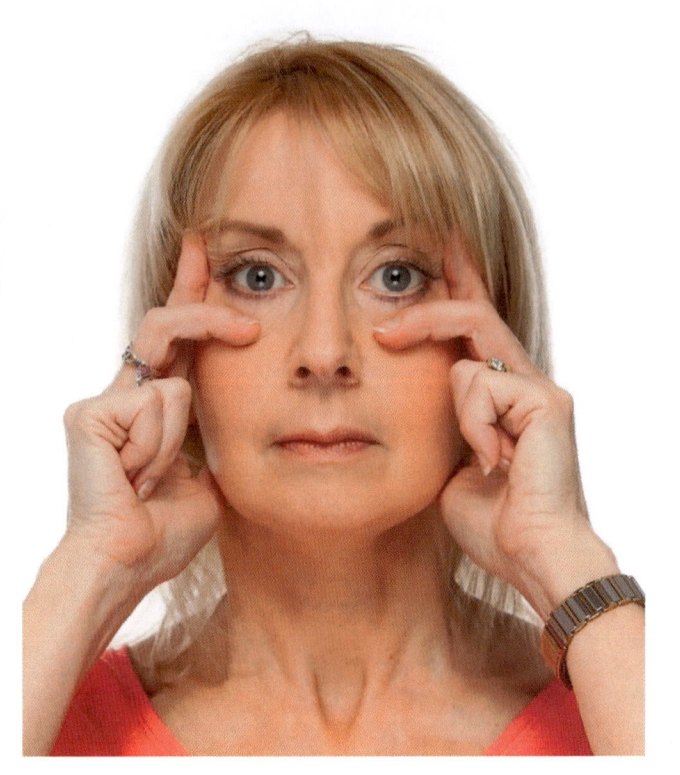

2. Contract (or squint) up with only the lower eyelids so you can feel the tiny muscles working in the bottom lid. Hold in this position for a second, concentrate on the muscle, then release it.

3. Repeat the contract, hold and release 5 times, concentrating on the lower lid muscle each time.

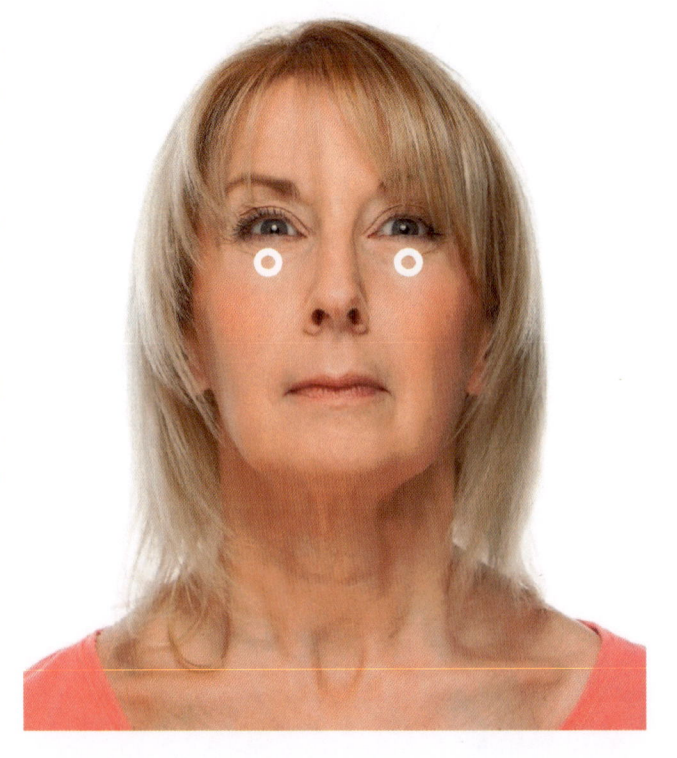

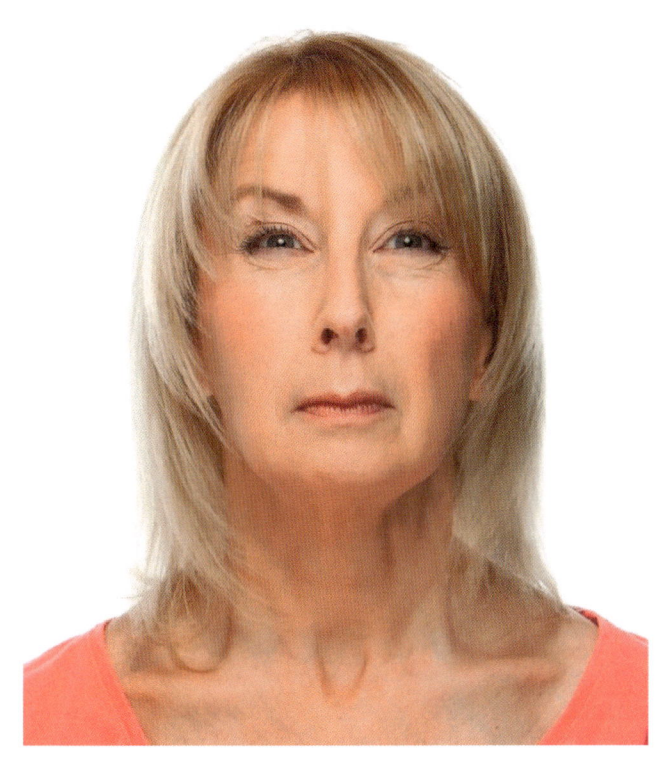

4. On the fifth squint up, start to squeeze the lower lid harder so that you can feel all the muscles under the eye working, right down to the top of the cheek. Check in the mirror and relax the top lid, nose, forehead or wherever other muscles are trying to help.

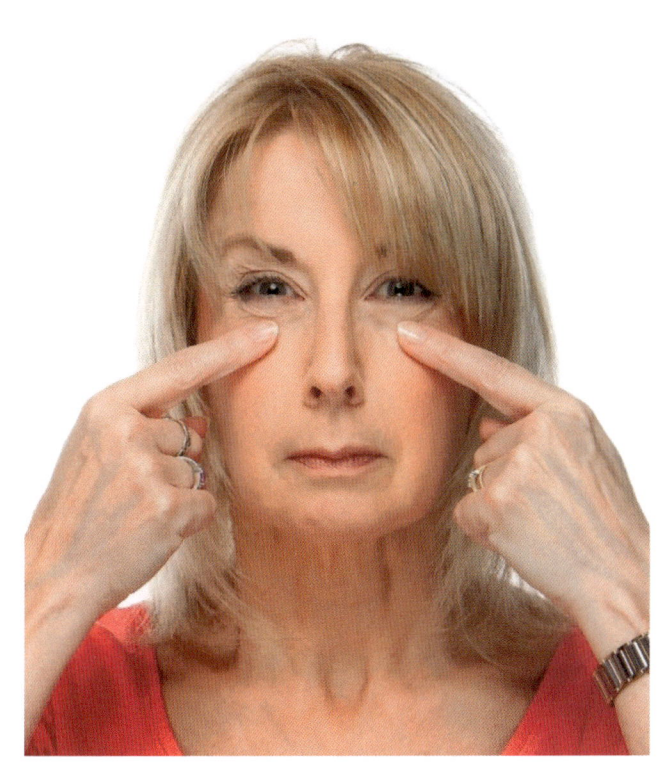

5. If you can't feel the muscles moving, place a fingertip just below each lid so you can feel the muscles.
Check your mirror to make sure only the lower lid is moving and not your entire eye.

Hold for a slow count of 10, or 15 seconds.

Relax and repeat 5 times. Only repeat this exercise 2 or 3 times in the first week.

Exercise 8: Eye Toner Two

Focus Point: The curve that forms the upper eye socket

Good for: brightening the eyes, hooded lids, crow's feet, lines and wrinkles, tired looking eyes, flat and drooping eyebrows.

Time: 2.30 minutes

Benefits
Eye Toner Two lifts away loose skin and completely reshapes the upper eye area. Results come quickly with this exercise! The upper lash line is enhanced: lashes appear more curved as the eyes open wider. Skin under the brow tightens and lifts to reveal the bone structure, right from the inside corner to the outer edge of the top lid. Crows' feet, drooping skin and expression lines all reduce as the skin tones for a fresher, brighter appearance. Improvements in circulation brighten the eyes themselves.

Muscles Worked
Orbicularis oculi, corrugator supercilii, depressor supercillii, procerus, frontalis, galea aponeurotica, occipitalis, posterior auricular.

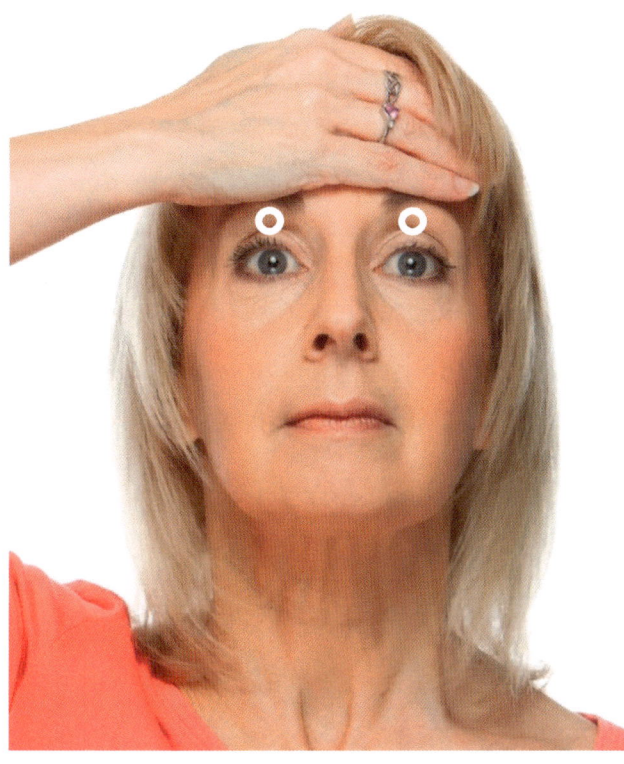

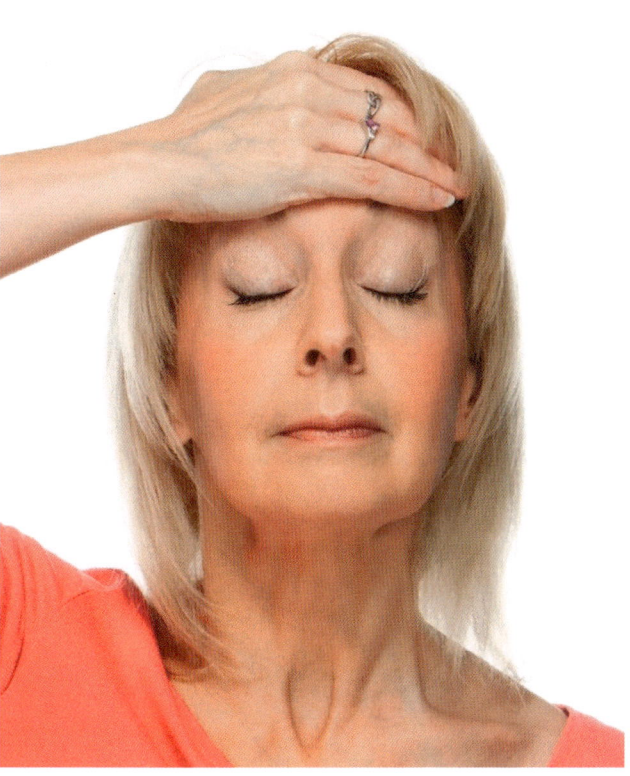

1. Sit straight and place an open palm lightly on the forehead as shown.

2. Lift the brows up and use the palm to smooth out forehead lines.

3. Lift brows up more, until there is a gentle stretch around the upper eye socket.

4. Close your eyes. Gently close the top lid more tightly. Don't put too much effort in: muscles are very delicate here.

5. Keep pulling the brows up and the top lids down all the way through.

6. Don't squeeze your eyelids shut or screw up the lower lids at all. It's a small, gentle movement.

Hold for a slow count of 10, or 15 seconds.

Relax and repeat 5 times.

Exercise 9: Chin and Jaw Toner

Focus Point: the middle centre of the neck – where the chin becomes the neck in the normal resting position

Good for: double chin, loose skin under the chin, 'turkey neck', jowls and marionette lines.

Time: 3.30 minutes

Benefits
This exercise on YouTube has millions of hits. It is a really great exercise to slim and tone double chins, and reduce flabbiness and loose skin – otherwise known as 'turkey neck'. If you've lost a definite jawline; this exercise will tone and firm, helping to remove jowls and marionette lines.

Muscles Worked
Platysma, anterior and posterior digastric, medial and lateral pterygoid, hyoid musculature. Neck muscles: sternocleidomastoid, semispinalis, splenis and longtissimus capitis, trapezius.

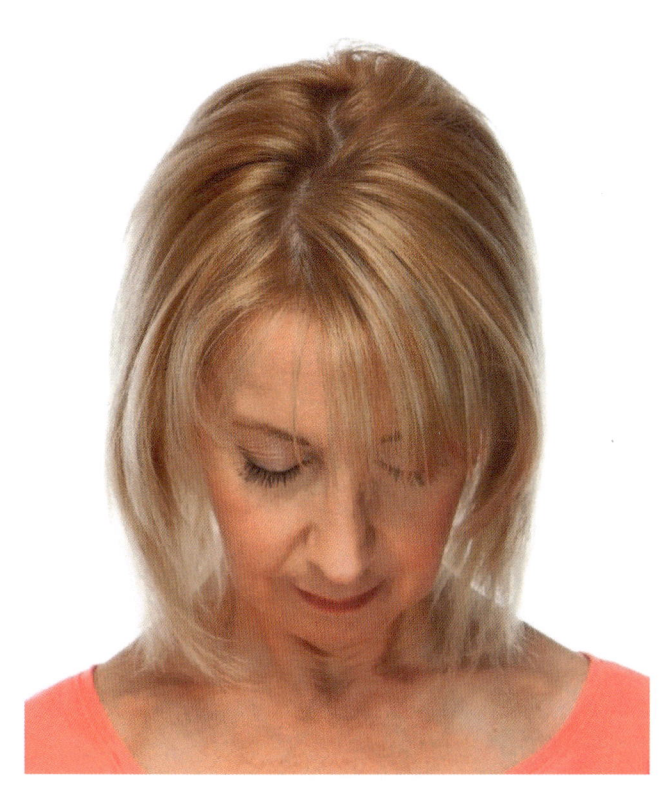

1. Drop your chin down to wherever is comfortable to feel a gentle stretch in the back of your neck. Relax your shoulders.

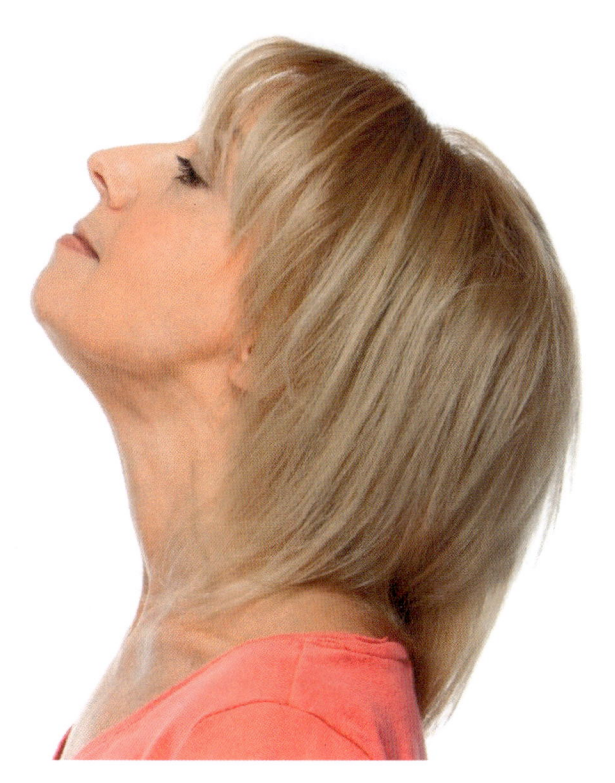

2. Lift the chin up, sit tall again, and raise your chin without straining.

3. Roll your lower jaw forward very slightly: no more than half an inch, to engage the muscles under the chin. You should feel the stretch under your chin, but no tension in the lower jaw, teeth, or the joint under your ear.

4. Hold for a count of 10.

5. Next, slowly lower your chin three inches, and then lift again, keeping the movement slow and even, particularly as you lower your chin.

6. Repeat the lifting and lowering 20 times, keep your head straight and your shoulders relaxed.

There should be no tension or discomfort in the main jaw joint under the ears. If there is, the lower jaw is pushed out too far. Roll it back in a little. Likewise, your neck should feel comfortable and sitting straight will prevent the upper cervical vertebrae from tension.

7. As you lower your chin for the last time, drop it back down to the starting position to gently stretch the back of the neck.

Repeat two or three times.

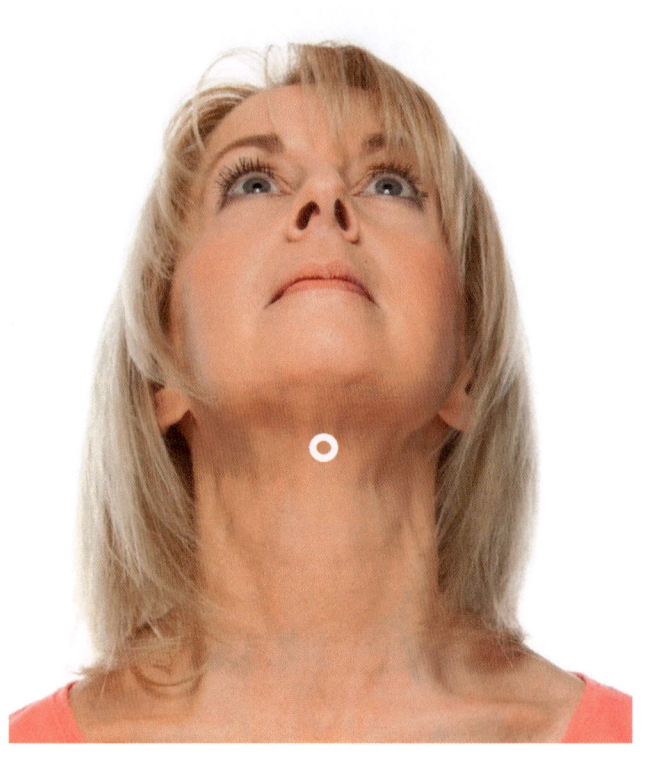

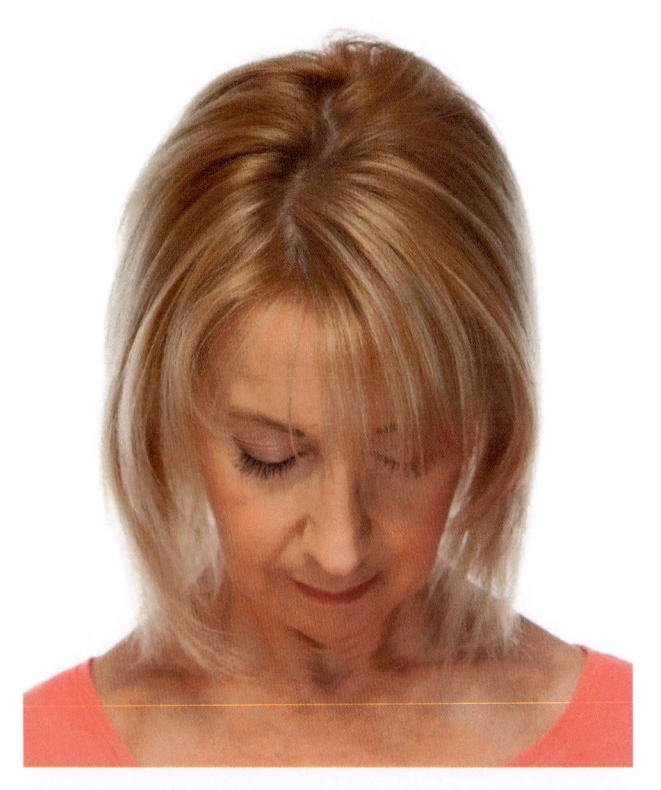

Exercise 10: Cheek Toner Two

Focus Point: the upper third of the cheek

Good for: adding volume to cheeks, under eye hollows, eye bags, shadows, flat, tired looking skin, lines and wrinkles and crow's feet.

Time: 3 minutes

Benefits

Cheek Toner Two targets the area where the first signs of ageing often show: the top half of the cheek. It rebuilds the lower lid and the entire upper cheek, including the outer corner of the eye. Muscles are gently built up to cushion the top of the cheek to give a natural curve. The skin plumps from underneath as the tissues strengthen. Lines and wrinkles reduce; skin looks smoother as it drapes properly over the area. Contours improve over the front and sides of the face as the balance is gently readjusted, for a healthy, toned and rejuvenated appearance.

This exercise combines the movements for Cheek Toner One and Eye Toner One to very effectively target the top of the cheek: often a difficult place to tone up.

Muscles Worked

Orbicularis oculi (lower and outer section), zygomaticus major and minor, buccinator, lateral pterygoid, risorius.

1. Keep your chin level. Place index fingers vertically alongside your eyes. Now place the middle fingers across, just under the lower lid. Check the photos and the position in your mirror and adjust if need be to smooth out potential wrinkling.

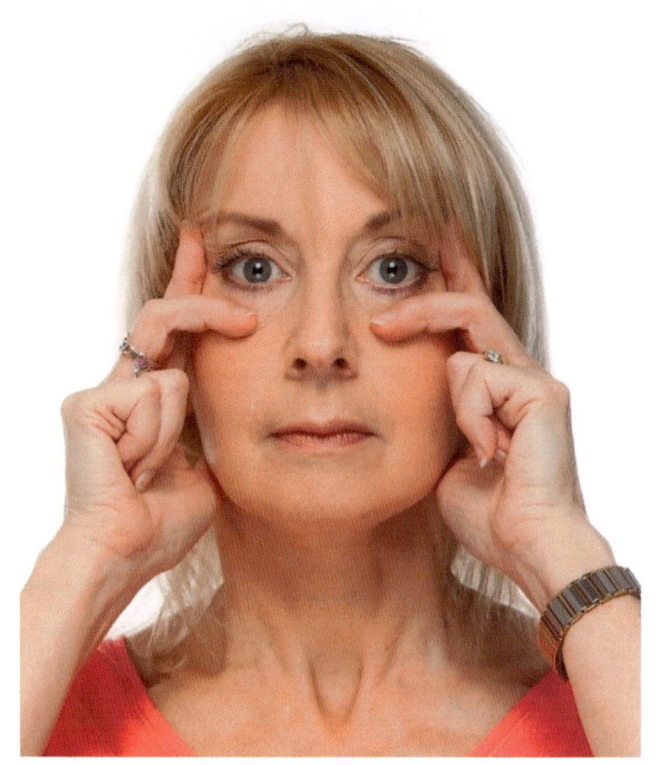

2. Contract your lower eyelid into a squint, as in Eye Toner One. Keep your top lids relaxed and open and don't screw your eyes up: they will try!

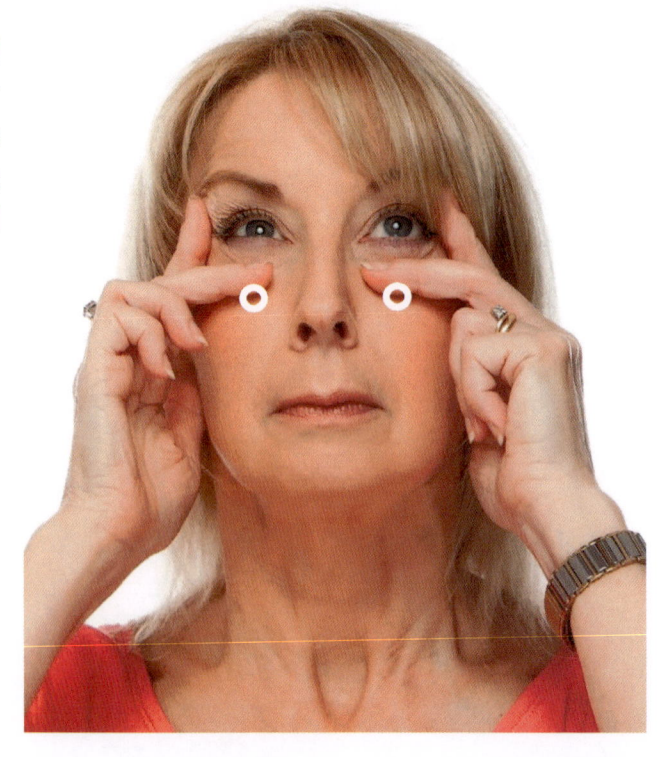

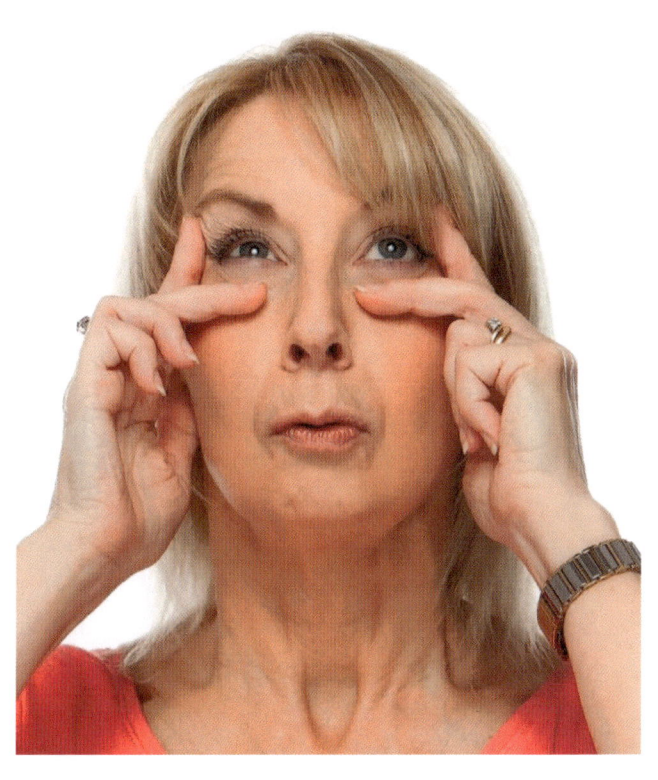

3. Open the mouth into a small pout with a little gap in between.

If it's easier to contract the lower eyelids and then pout, swap points 3 and 5.

4. Use your mirror and adjust the finger positions if any of the lines are not smoothed out during the exercise.

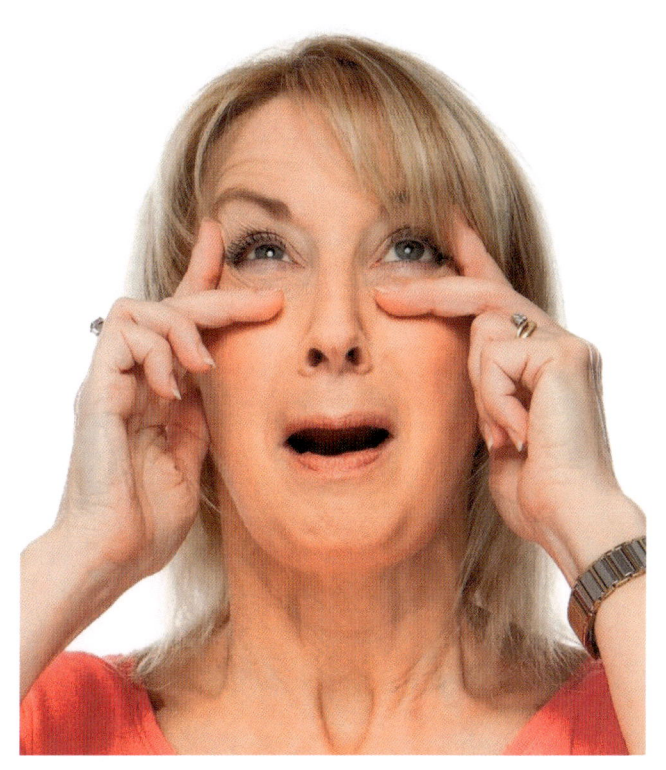

5. Lift the top lip into a smile with your mouth open.

6. Keep pushing the cheeks to work hard throughout, all the while using only the cheeks and under the eyes. Keep the lower jaw, upper lid and forehead relaxed.

Hold for a slow count of 10, or 15 seconds.

Relax and repeat 5 times.

Exercise 11: Mouth Area Shaper

Focus Point: either side of the mouth where the stretch is hardest.

Good for: mouth, lips, jowls, the entire lower face, softened jawline, chin, marionette and naso-labial lines.

Time: 2.20 minutes

Benefits
This is a fabulous exercise for the lower face. First, it erases deep naso-labial folds either side of the mouth by lifting excess skin away. It also tones and reshapes the lips, and the area each side of the mouth without adding bulk. As the muscles tone, the heaviness that is a feature of older faces disappears: revealing a neater and slimmer lower face. It lifts and reduces marionette lines and jowls, and finally, firms and defines the chin and jawline.

We have a huge amount of enquiries about jowls, marionette lines and general softening of the face around the jaw. It is because of gravity that our faces sag with age. It can take about 4-5 months with the recommended program to see results here, because the muscles in the top half of the cheek have to lift away first. Once the cheek muscles are sitting up where they should be, you will be able to see the results further down.

The good news is that the lower face will continue to tone and neaten way past the 3 month intensive phase. Even doing Faceworks 3 times a week is enough to keep improving the area, and this exercise is a really easy one to do anywhere.

Muscles Worked
Orbicularis oris, depressor anguli oris, mentalis, depressor labii inferioris, levator labii superioris, zygomaticus major and minor, risorius, nasalis, lateral pterygoid.

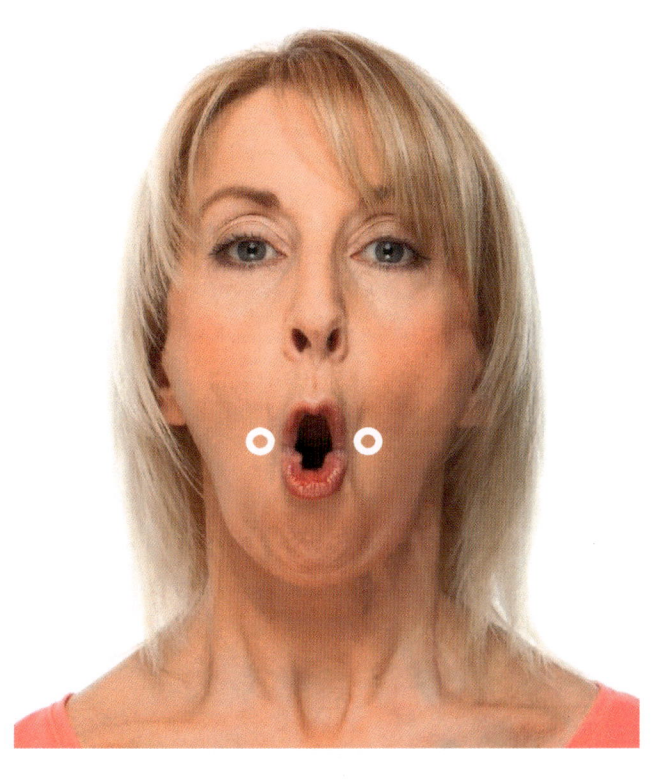

1. Keep your chin level. Open your lips into the longest, narrowest 'O':

The easiest way is to open your mouth and then bring the sides in towards each other, as if you're trying to touch the lips together lengthways.

2. Don't drive the exercise with the lower jaw; the movement is with the lips only.

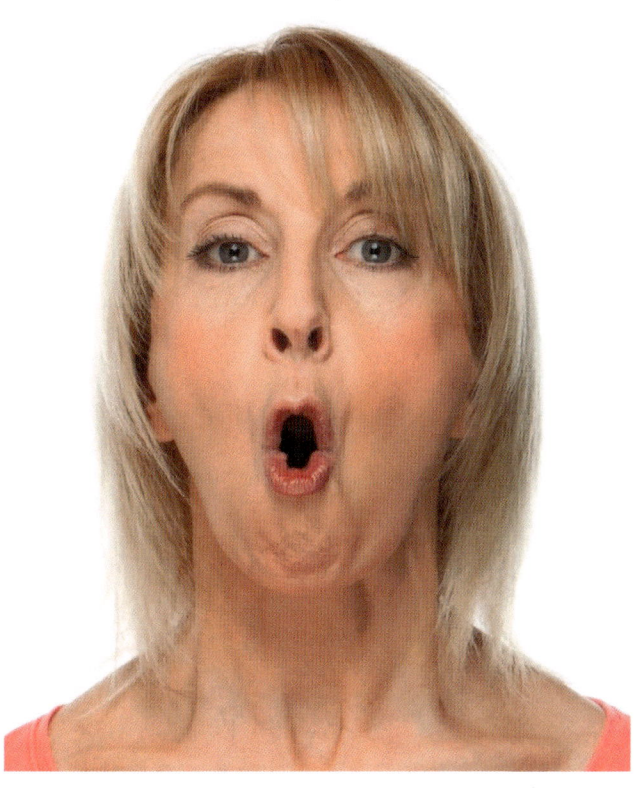

3. Try to increase the length of the 'O': pushing the lips forward can help.

You will feel the tautness both sides of your mouth and this is the place to concentrate on – keep the effort up all the way through.

Hold for a slow count of 10, or 15 seconds.

Relax and repeat 5 times.

Exercise 12: Face Finisher

Focus Point: the lips – keep the open and close movements slow and even

Good for: improving circulation in muscles and skin, a healthy-looking complexion.

Time: 1.45 minutes

Benefits
This is a great exercise to finish your workout. It continues the toning effect of the previous exercise on the lower face and mouth. The biggest benefit is due to the continuous opening and closing: boosting the circulation of blood and lymph to leave your skin glowing. The lymph fluid removes toxins from tissues and an efficient lymph flow is very important for the health of your skin. The exercises help to normalise skin problems and increase the health of skin naturally. Healthy skin means fewer wrinkles later on.

Muscles Worked
All lower face and jaw muscles.

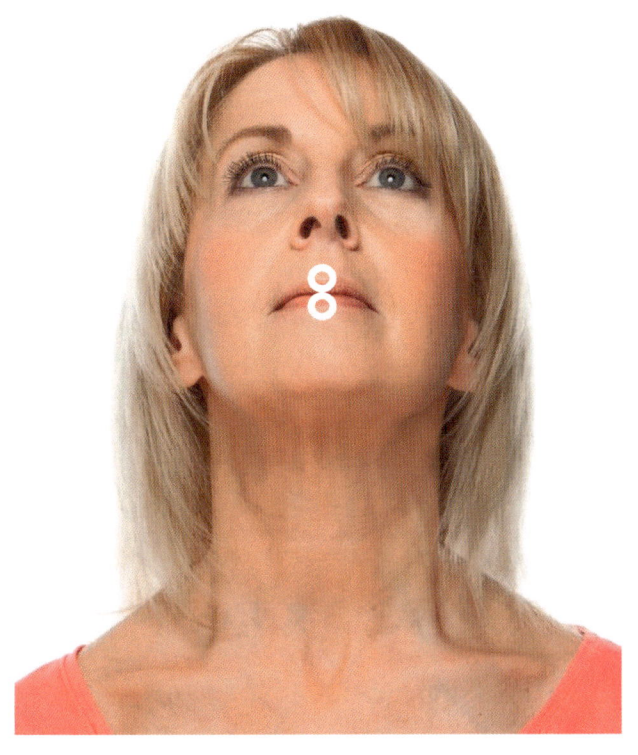

This exercise is a continuous sequence: it doesn't relax and repeat.

1. Sit straight, with the chin lifted slightly.

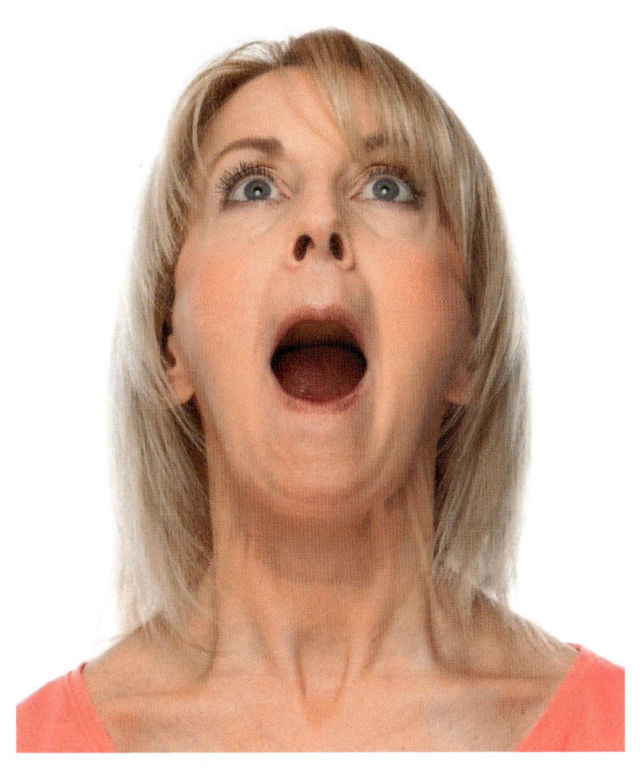

2. Open your mouth slowly and deliberately as big an 'O' as possible, without straining your jaw.

Hold for a second.

3. Close again slowly, bringing the lips round to close into a small 'O'. Hold for a second in this position.

4. Repeat opening and closing the mouth 20 times. Keep the movement slow and even, concentrating on the shape your lips make as they open and close.

5. Relax.

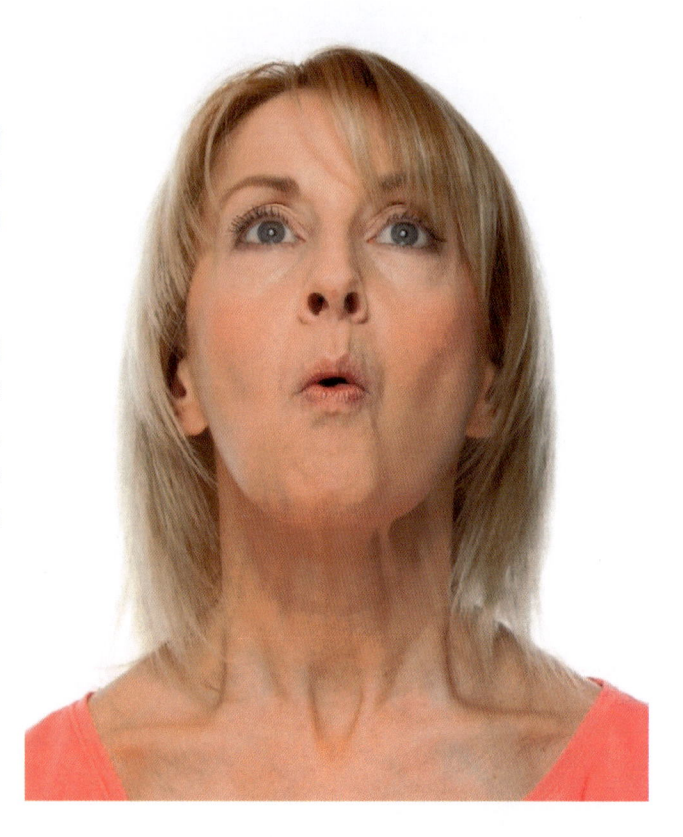

Relaxing Massage

Do this quick and effective self-massage at the beginning or end of your Faceworks session. It is great to relieve stress and fatigue, or whenever you need a 5 minute break.

- With both hands, feel up the centre back of the neck towards the base of the skull. Feel for the area where the back of the neck meets the skull. Massage gently with the fingertips using a comfortable but firm pressure in the centre then work your way up onto the base of the skull. Make slow, deep, circular movements with the fingertips, taking care to massage thoroughly wherever it feels sore. Gradually work your way out along the base of the skull until you reach the back of the ears.

- Next, cup the right hand around the back of the sneck and massage the cervical (neck) vertebrae on the side where your fingers are. Use as much pressure as is comfortable, working up and down the back of the neck along the spine; again using slow, deep circular movements. Swap hands and use your left hand to massage the right side.

- Place the tip of your thumb on the skull at the top your ear where it inserts into your skull; and place the remaining fingertips on the head, 3 inches further up and slightly spread out. Massage with your fingertips and move your hand in an arc so that the fingers cover a semi-circle round the skull above the ear, all the while using your thumb as the pivot. Increase the strength of the pressure to whatever is comfortable for you. The area is often very sore, so be gentle but thorough!

- Place the fingertips back in the starting position from before and with a quick, firm pressure, 'pinch' the thumb and fingers together in an arc around the ear. This movement is a kinesiology technique that releases the temporalis muscles: often the cause of tension headaches and that 'tight' feeling around the head we get when stressed.

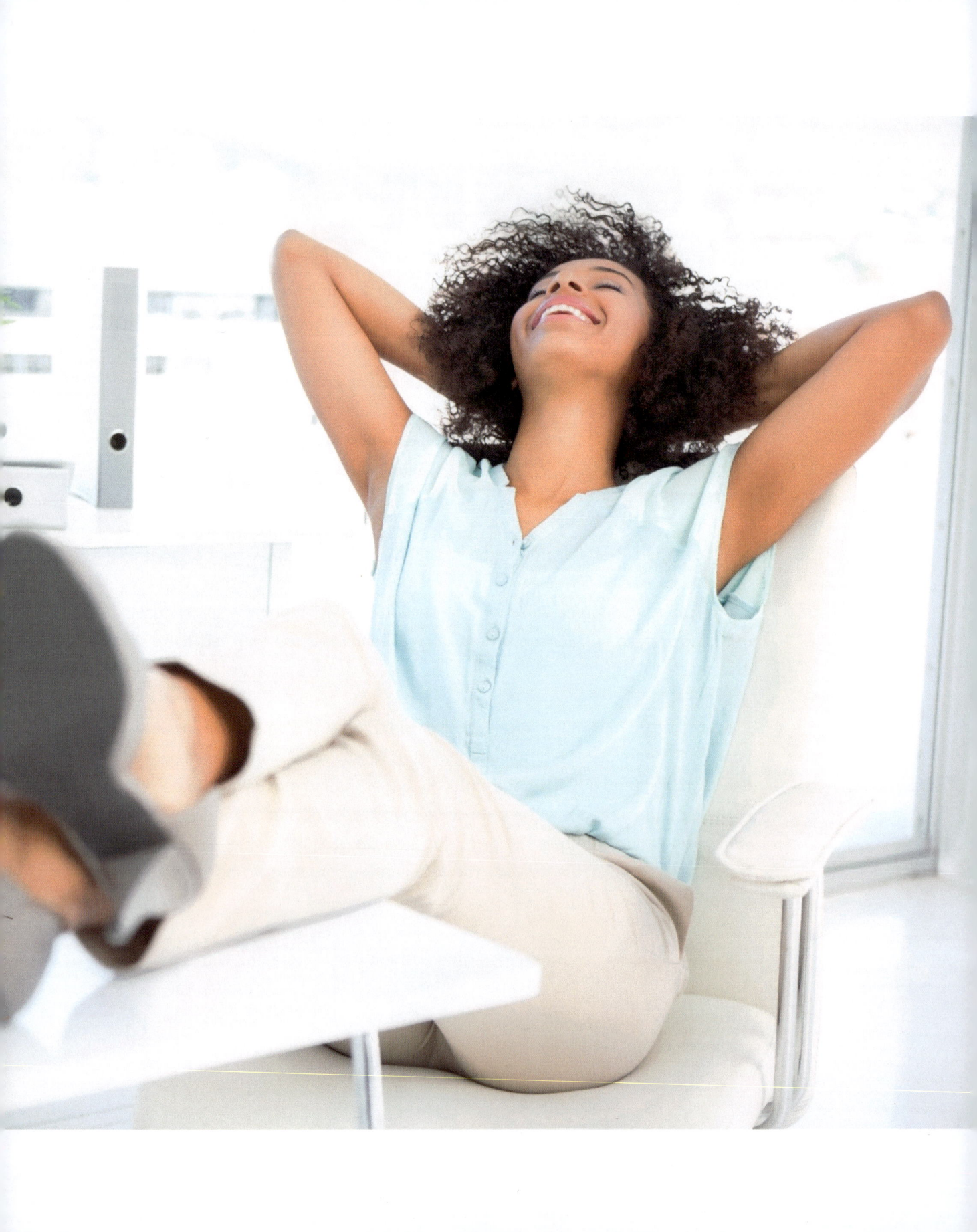

- Next, place fingertips along the hairline, slightly spread out. Massage in small circular movements to release and relax the frontalis muscle. Work along the hairline towards the temples.

- Repeat the massage along the top of your eyebrows, from the centre out to the ends. Be gentle here, as the eyebrow ridge can also be very sore!

- Now move the massage down to the jaw: start an inch below the front of the ears and around where the 'corner' of the jaw is. Feel for tight and sore places, gently moving your fingers into the dips and hollows to release tension.

- Finally, shut your eyes and place your cupped palms over them. Don't use any pressure at all. You should feel the gentle warmth from your palms gradually seep into your eyelids, eyes, and the muscles behind your eyes. Concentrate on the warmth: you may feel a tingling sensation in your hands or your eyes as the tissues relax. We all have a natural healing ability: that's why we use touch to comfort others. It is rare to use the healing touch on ourselves, but it is instantly nurturing. Hold this position for a minimum of two minutes. This is really refreshing for eye strain, or if you spend long periods on a computer.

When our muscles hold tension, the fibres can become used to a higher resting tone than is usual, and it can take a while for them to fully release and relax. Feeling tired or yawning after the massage is a good sign that the muscles are releasing.

Questions and Problems

Pain

Faceworks is carefully designed to be safe and should not cause anything greater than a manageable muscle ache during the workout. If you have any health or structural problems it is wise to get approval from your doctor or specialist before you try Faceworks. The most common query is jaw pain, which can occur when the jaw is pushed out too far, for example in Exercise 9: the Chin and Jaw Toner.

None of the exercises have extreme movement and if you are finding that your face, neck or your jaw hurts significantly after your workout, stop exercising and see your doctor. If they are happy for you to carry on, wait until the pain goes before restarting. Review the positions and reduce the movements. Remember to be precise with the positions, face muscles are a lot smaller than body muscles. They will tone up without using brute force.

Pain or Headaches from Over-active Muscles

Pain can be caused by facial muscles that refuse to relax. Over-active muscles cause headaches and a feeling of pressure or tightness in a number of places on the skull. Most commonly this is across the eyebrows, on the forehead, over the top of the head, or around the back of the ears. Being under too much pressure in life equals pressure in the body. If headaches are persistent, get them checked.

Over active muscles are often those associated with the jaw, at the hairline or over the scalp. Pain in the temples and around the ear is caused by the temporo-mandibular joint. Pain at the hairline and over the scalp is caused by the frontalis muscle on the forehead, and/or the occipitalis at the back of the scalp. The frontalis and occipitalis are connected by a wide, sheet-like tendon that covers the top of the head.

Since all these places are sites that get tight from stress, adding exercise to an already over-active muscle can cause pain. Check if the muscles are at a higher resting tone than they should be by using the Relaxing Massage. Use it before or after your workout. If regular use of the massage doesn't ease things off, it may be worth looking at the balance of your life to see where that tension is potentially coming from.

Poor Results

During the time I've been involved with facial exercise, a failure to get results is down to something vital being missed. Whether that 'something vital' is not following the 'How To', not working the muscles correctly, not working out enough, or even not being able to see the changes in yourself – the solution to all of them is time. Take time to read the chapters you might have skimmed over before, take time to read the steps to do the exercises, take time to do the workout, or time to sit and really look at - and appreciate - yourself.

In a practical sense poor results can be solved by one of the following:

Poor Results (1)

Your face hasn't changed at all, and you don't feel an ache in the muscles during the exercises or after your workout session.

The reason is that the muscles are not being worked enough to tone up. The next time you do your workout, check where the Focus Point is (the white circles on the photos show where these are) and follow each step carefully.

After you have the position right, the next vital step is working the muscles. To say that another way: when you 'hold' for 15 seconds, carry on doing the movement you made to put the face into the position it's in. If the instruction is to lift the brows up, *keep lifting them up* for 15 seconds. The only thing that makes a muscle tone up is working it harder than normal. There should be a noticeable ache in the Focus Point muscles during each repetition.

Check the time each repetition is held for too: 15 seconds is the right amount of time.

Poor Results (2)

Your face feels like it is being worked but the results aren't noticeable

When you do your workout, check if other parts of your face are moving or scrunching up, for example your forehead on the Cheek Toners, or your mouth for the eye exercises. If other parts of your face are 'helping', then the muscles that should be driving the exercise can't work properly: no matter how much effort you put in.

To work the right muscles, put your fingertips on the Focus Point on every exercise and use *only* those muscles to contract or squeeze. Some of the muscles; such as those around the eye, are tiny and you won't see them contracting. It's necessary to isolate and work specific muscles properly for your face to change, and using the Focus Point like this should instantly feel more effective.

Plateau

The exercises work to begin with, but stop giving results after a while. This occurs because: very honestly, you stop concentrating. Basically, you know the exercises well, but **because** you know them, your concentration drops off a little. Then the muscles stop working so hard – and the results stop coming.

The solution is to pretend that you're learning the exercises again. Go back to basics and follow the instructions with a mirror: really concentrate on the Focus Point. When you think the muscles are pushed as far as they can go, push them a little more.

New Lines and Wrinkles

New lines occur when the movements are too aggressive and exaggerated. You'll notice on the photos that even in position for the exercise, the movements aren't excessive and the skin remains mainly smooth.

The first thing to do is use a mirror to see which exercises are causing the lines to form. Check the position of the exercise and adjust it if isn't right. If your face isn't scrunching or moving where it shouldn't, smooth the lines out with your fingertips as you exercise. If it isn't possible to smooth the lines out, leave the exercise(s) out.

Will all the loose skin and sagging lift?

For a person aged 40-50 who is ageing at an average rate, 80% or more of the sagging and loose skin should disappear. If you are older than this, you will still have excellent results, though some loose skin may remain. Results depend on the elasticity of your skin and its' biological (rather than actual) age, and also if you're through menopause. We get overjoyed testimonials from people in their 60s and 70s, and it's obvious that a little loose skin doesn't detract from the overall facelift.

Will all my lines and wrinkles go away?

Lines and wrinkles physically reduce by 30 - 40%, and because of the improvements in the structure of your face, they'll appear to reduce by around 50%. Many lines are a combination of a line plus sagging skin: when the sagging lifts, lines can almost vanish. A major benefit of exercising is that new lines form more slowly because the condition of your skin is improved. The condition of skin is affected by many external and internal influences: hormones, weight loss or gain, stress, vitamin or mineral deficiency, diet, hydration, gut health, pollution, and the weather, to name a few. The e-mails we have about skin worries frequently flag up stress as a major factor.

Why does my face look different just after I have done Faceworks?

The exercises increase the blood supply to the face and neck. Because muscles work harder, they need more oxygen and glucose. The increase in circulation causes facial tissue to become plumper for a short time after doing the workout. This is beneficial for all layers of the skin, as cell renewal and repair become more efficient. Improvements to the complexion are usually the first changes noted.

Can I do more than 5 workouts a week?

The recommended schedule of 5 times a week means it fits easily into most people's schedule. It isn't necessary to do more than this. It is, however, safe to do more should you want to. Begin on 5 times a week for the first month, go on to 6 and finally 7 times a week. Add the extra workouts over a period of 2 or 3 weeks to allow your facial muscles to adapt.

Some people aim for two workouts a day, though this isn't needed long term. Again, work up slowly and pay close attention to how your muscles are feeling. The muscles need time to recuperate and it is best to **leave at least 6 hours** between workouts: perhaps one workout in the morning, and a second in the evening. The second workout can be a full one or a smaller set, e.g. one of the ready-made Mini Workouts, or choose a couple of extras for your personal 'problem' areas. Check the Quick Lists to find some.

Can the muscles be built up too much?

Faceworks won't overdevelop your face. Muscles build gradually and the fibres within the muscle rebuild to a limited size, so you won't look like you've had too many fillers, or look unnatural. The workouts carefully rebuild for a natural, balanced result and it isn't possible for your face to build up like a bodybuilder's.

Can I have Botox or Fillers while doing Faceworks?

People do use the exercises after having fillers or Botox, though I'm unable to guarantee or advise on the effects or results. Your first contact should always be with the professional who carries out the procedure. You should ask if the procedure is compatible with facial exercise. For Botox, it is possible that any kind of facial exercise may shorten the length of time that the chemical is active. In the case of fillers, you should ask if facial exercise will cause the substance to move or change in any way. Both these types of procedures are beyond my field of expertise.

Can I do Faceworks after surgery?

Again, please contact your surgeon for their professional opinion on the suitability of Faceworks after any surgery, whether dental, cosmetic or health related.

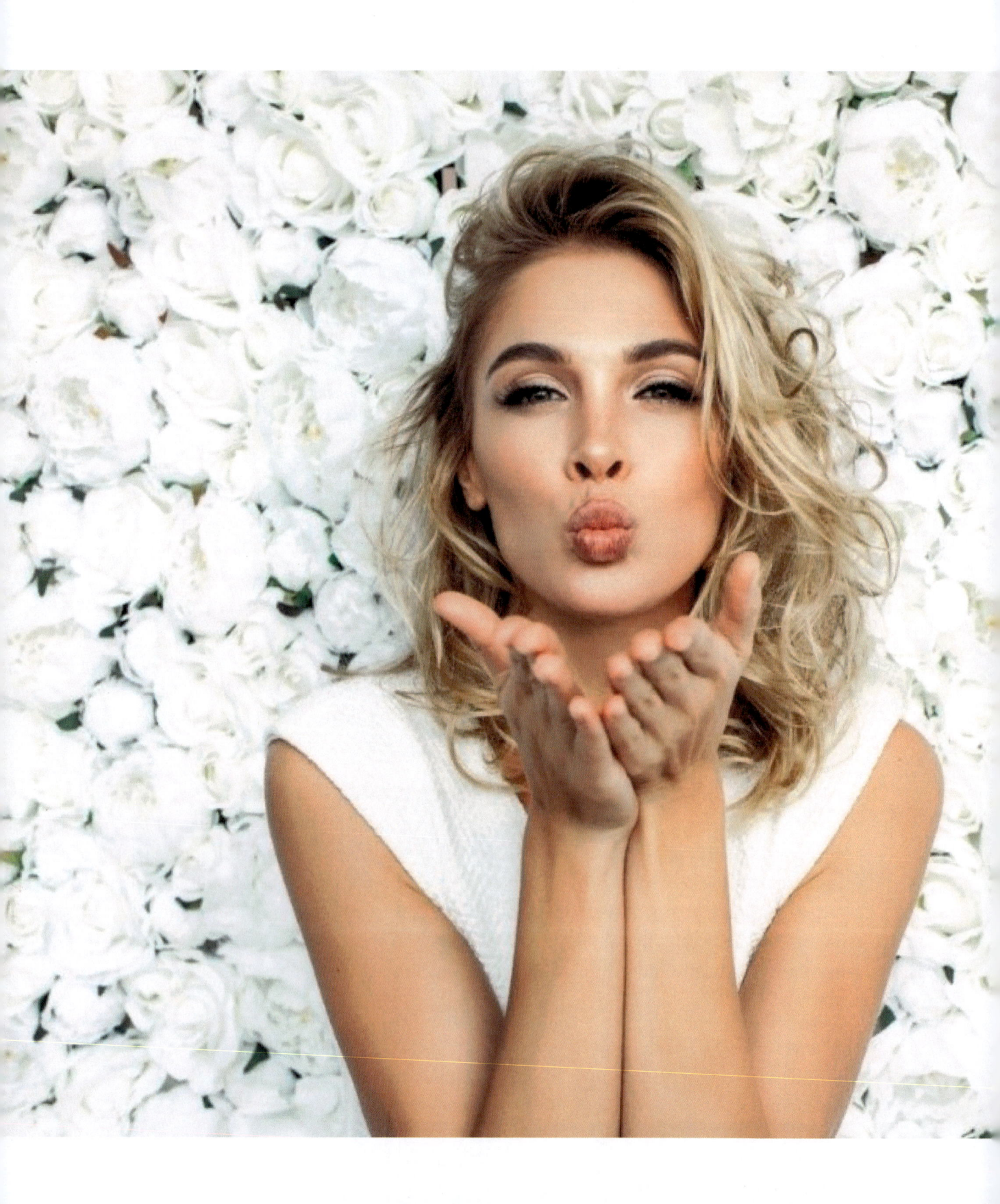

The Express Workout

The Express workout is a less intense full face workout and it's is a good alternative if you're time-poor. I originally did this for a very busy guy who wanted a workout he could do in his lunch hour. It's ideal for the 35-45 age group who are noticing the first general signs of ageing. Use this workout if you don't have much sagging, but want an overall 'revive and tone' to freshen your face and complexion.

The schedule is the same as the Complete Workout, with one 15 minute workout on 5 days a week for the first 3 months. After 3 months the schedule is 2 workouts to maintain, or up to 4 times a week to boost results more.

Express Workout time: 15 minutes

Exercise List

3. Mouth Shaper Two

6. Cheek Toner One

7. Eye Toner One

8. Eye Toner Two

11. Mouth Area Shaper

12. Face Finisher

Ways to use the Express Workout
- With a regular 5 times a week schedule, the same as the Complete Workout.
- As a gentle introduction to the Complete Workout. Use the Express Workout for two weeks before going on to the Complete Workout.
- If you're not sure if face exercises are for you, try this workout first.
- Swap with the Complete Workout on days when you don't have much time.

The Instant Boosters: Your Secret Weapon

The exercises in the Express Workout have another great benefit. Each one gives an instant boost and leave you looking refreshed, like you've had an instant facial. No-one will ever know about the late night you had, or that you're feeling less than 100%. The immediate effects are caused by an increase in blood circulation into the muscles and deep skin layers, and they'll have you glowing and gorgeous in minutes.

Ways to use the Instant Boosters:
- Choose the ones you need for an instant fix: just eyes, just skin, just lips - one, three or all six.
- Use them if you look tired or don't feel 100% to get you back to your best.
- They are brilliant to use as a beauty treatment before an evening out.
- To sharpen mental clarity and awareness: useful for work, or as a quick pick-me-up.

Using the six exercises like this instantly brightens, and gives a little 'plump and enhance' for about half an hour, sometimes longer. The increase in circulation is particularly good for clearing fatigue around the eyes and improving mental function.

The Mini Workouts

These four little workouts are great to use if you only have one area you'd like to lift. Another option is to use them to intensify results for problem areas, either as a second workout during the first 12 weeks, or post-12 weeks to maintain your facelift.

At just 10 minutes the Mini workouts give a swift boost for the places that need a little more exercise to stay lifted. If you 're using only these, the schedule once again is a workout 5 days a week, the same as the other workouts. They are all available with videos on the website.

Brow and Eye Lift Mini Workout
Workout Time: 10 minutes

Exercise List

1. Facial Warm-up

5. Eyebrow Lift

7. Eye Toner One

8. Eye Toner Two

A quick lift and tone for the delicate brow and eye area. The gentle toning action of the exercises gives a fast pick-me-up when you look tired, or feel weary. This workout targets flat or low eyebrows, frown lines, sagging, crow's feet, wrinkles and puffiness.

Cheek Boost Mini Workout
Workout Time: 12 minutes

Exercise List

1. Facial Warm-up

2. Mouth Shaper One

6. Cheek Toner One

10. Cheek Toner Two

This little cheek workout boosts results over the cheeks and increases natural contouring on the sides of the face. It also targets the common under-eye problems of dark circles, puffiness, eye bags and deep tear troughs.

Lip and Mouth Mini Workout

Workout Time: 10 minutes

Exercise List

1. Facial Warm-up

3. Mouth Shaper Two

4. Lip Builder

11. Mouth Area Shaper

This is a fast workout that plumps the lips and lifts the mouth area. The exercises reduce lines and folds around the mouth, giving naturally lovely lips and a defined mouth with neater, smoother surrounding area. For thin lips, drooping mouth corners, smile or laugh lines and naso-labial folds.

Chin and Jawline Mini Workout

Workout Time - 10 minutes

Exercise List

1. Facial Warm-up

2. Mouth Shaper One

9. Chin and Jaw Toner

11. Mouth Area Shaper

If you're under 40, the Chin and Jawline Mini Workout may be all you'll need for the lower face. It's great to reduce double chins, slim the look of plump faces and to give contours along the jawline. You'll see results around the mouth with smoother skin and a reduction in deep expression lines.

For more general sagging over the lower face, use the Complete Workout to start with, and either add this as a second workout, or use it after you've got your facelift.

Quick List 1: Effects and Results

Use the list below as a quick guide to find the effects and results achievable for each exercise. Generally, exercises for the top half of the face lift, tone and rebuild muscle, while those for the lower half of the face lift, tone and streamline. This ensures that the shape of the face tones appropriately to enhance the natural balance.

In Quick List 2 you'll find the best exercises for your own problem areas. The Glossary of Terms to explain the not-so-familiar words can be found at the end of this book.

The Results and Effects of Each Exercise

Exercise 1: Facial Warm Up
Based on the yoga 'Lion' asana, this exercise warms and tones muscles in the face, lips, jaw and neck in preparation for specific exercises. It stimulates blood flow in the entire face, skin and neck, including the throat muscles and endocrine glands.

Exercise 2: Mouth Shaper One
Mouth Shaper One plumps lips, lifts the mouth corners and reduces the naso-labial fold that runs from the nose to each side of the mouth. It tones deep jaw muscles, and builds the surface muscles of the cheek area, improving cheek contours, and tones muscles under the chin.

Exercise 3: Mouth Shaper Two
This exercise plumps the lips, enhances the shape and stops lips looking flat and thin. It softens expression lines around the mouth, and vertical lines in the top lip. The mouth area is plumped and filled out, especially from under the nose to the mouth. Lastly, it increases blood circulation in the nose tip.

Exercise 4: Lip Builder
The Lip Builder plumps and enlarges the lip profile; especially the cupids' bow, which tends to flatten with age. It also tones the muscles either side of the nose.

Exercise 5: Eyebrow Lift
This exercise lifts the entire brow and defines the arch to frame the eyes. Lifting the brow also lifts loose and drooping skin on the upper lid and eye corners. It erases frown ridges and heaviness between the brows. Finally, it tones the muscles over the top and at the back of the scalp for a general lifted effect.

Exercise 6: Cheek Toner One
The cheek contours are shaped, tightened and sculpted with this exercise, giving definition to the whole face. The muscles move up to sit on the cheekbone where they should be, giving the impression of higher cheekbones. As cheek muscles lift up, the lower cheek and the sides of the face are completely reshaped. This exercise builds volume in thin or flat cheeks, so restoring the correct width across the top of the cheek, and reducing weight at the bottom. It also adds definition to plump faces.

Exercise 7: Eye Toner One
This exercise tones and lifts loose skin and under-eye bags, and erases signs of tiredness. It builds up the flat or hollow area around the lower eye socket. Circulation around the delicate eye area is increased, which reduces puffiness and dark circles. The eyes are brighter with a more 'awake' look. The lash line is more defined; and as the skin plumps up, wrinkles are smoothed out.

Exercise 8: Eye Toner Two
Eye Toner Two tightens and tones the entire upper lid, lifting away excess skin, hooded lids, deep crows' feet and wrinkles. Eyes open up and look brighter; signs of tiredness are erased. Along the brows, frown ridges and deep lines smooth out. Finally, tension is eased in the eyes and scalp. Increased tone in muscles over the scalp gives a general lifted effect.

Exercise 9: Chin and Jaw Toner
This exercise is excellent for toning and lifting a double chin; reducing jowls, marionette lines and loose skin under the chin to give more definition to the entire jawline. The extremely gentle action of this exercise prevents neck tendons from becoming enlarged.

Exercise 10: Cheek Toner Two
This exercise lifts and shapes the upper cheek. It rebuilds the deep cheek muscles here, filling out under eye hollows to support and smooth the delicate skin. It also increases circulation to the under eye area to target puffiness, tear troughs, grooves and shadows.

Exercise 11: Mouth Area Shaper

This exercise tones and slims the entire lower face. It erases naso-labial folds (those troublesome folds of skin) that run from nose corners to mouth, so that mouth corners are lifted. It also targets marionette lines and jowls, by lifting and streamlining this often overlooked area. The lower face becomes neater and tidier as the entire weight of the face moves up.

Exercise 12: Face Finisher

The gentle stretching and contracting of this exercise improves lymph flow to effectively remove toxins that have built up during the workout, making this an ideal final exercise. It loosens tension in the temporo-mandibular joint: the jaw joint in front of the ear, and boosts circulation to the entire face.

Quick List 2: Your Personal Face Savers

Use this quick list to find the best exercises to fix stubborn problems. You might not need all the exercises listed. The idea here is to find one or two star performers; and either double up when you're working on your facelift, or use to prevent things dropping when your facelift is complete (even if you have zero time).

If you double up; do the additional exercises earlier or later in the day, not at the same time as the full workout.

Forehead and brows
For a heavy forehead, frown ridges or lines, flat or low eyebrows:

>Exercise 5: Eyebrow Lift
>Exercise 8: Eye Toner Two

Top eyelid
For hooded eyes, loose skin on the top lid, folds or deep wrinkles at outer corners:

>Exercise 5: Eyebrow Lift
>Exercise 7: Eye Toner One
>Exercise 8: Eye Toner Two

Eyes
For tired, or weary eyes, or to brighten up your peepers:

>Exercise 7: Eye Toner One
>Exercise 8: Eye Toner Two

Under eyes
For under-eye bags, dark shadows, puffiness, deep tear troughs and hollows, loose skin and wrinkles:

>Exercise 6: Cheek Toner One
>Exercise 7: Eye Toner One
>Exercise 8: Eye Toner Two
>Exercise 10: Cheek Toner Two

Cheeks

For flat and shapeless cheeks, chubby or heavy cheeks, sagging or loose skin, naso-labial folds and creases:

>Exercise 1: Facial Warm Up
>Exercise 2: Mouth Shaper One
>Exercise 6: Cheek Toner One
>Exercise 10: Cheek Toner Two
>Optional Exercise 11: Mouth Area Shaper

Mouth

For thin or small lips, drooping or hidden mouth corners, or vertical lines in the top lip:

>Exercise 2: Mouth Shaper One
>Exercise 3: Mouth Shaper Two
>Exercise 4: Lip Builder
>Exercise 11: Mouth Area Shaper

Leave out Exercise 4 if you have vertical lines on your lips.

Jawline

For marionette lines, jowls, a soft jawline, and heaviness around the jaw:

>Exercise 1: Facial Warm up
>Exercise 2: Mouth Shaper One
>Exercise 9: Chin and Jaw Toner
>Exercise 11: Mouth Area Shaper
>Optional: Exercise 6: Cheek Toner One

Chin and neck

For a double chin, loose skin under the chin and on the front of the neck:

>Exercise 1: Facial Warm Up,
>Exercise 2: Mouth Shaper One
>Exercise 9: Chin and Jaw Toner
>Optional: Exercise 11: Mouth Area Shaper

Skin

For dull or tired-looking skin, spots and breakouts, dryness, uneven skin tone, blotchiness, or redness:

    Exercise 1: Facial Warm Up
    Exercise 6: Cheek Toner One
    Exercise 11: Mouth Area Shaper
    Exercise 12: Face Finisher

Part Three

The Science of Facial Exercise

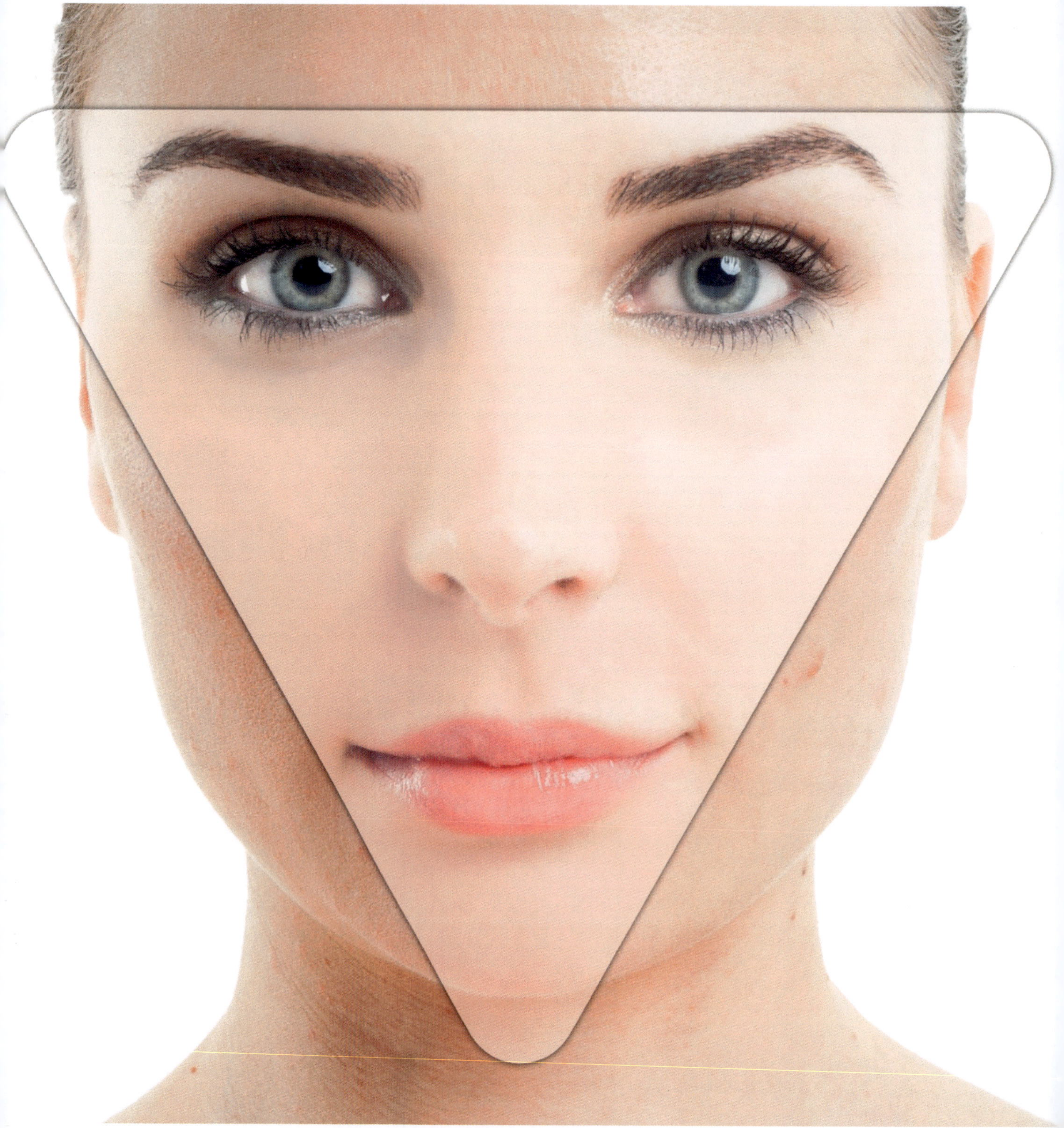

The Science of Facial Exercise

My grandmother thought the idea of exercise; or 'physical jerks' as she called it, was hilarious. My mother thought I was beyond mad to **choose** to use weights; run, or exert myself for the sake of keeping fit, and both of them happily accepted the 'inevitable' decline of their bodies into premature old age. Both spent their final years almost completely bedridden.

We're a lot more aware than past generations about the need to work our bodies to keep healthy and mobile to enjoy life to the full as we get older. We all know that the right exercise makes our bodies healthier, leaner and stronger. The added extra is being fit tends to make people look younger too. Exercise is a science, and Faceworks applies that science to the face. The program gives you the right exercises to look younger and healthier- whatever age you are. In this section we'll look at how and why facial exercise works so well.

The Right Facial Balance

Faceworks has been developed with professional knowledge of anatomy and physiology. The exercises are specifically designed to enhance and to restore; and then maintain, the best proportions for your face. The exercises for the top half of the face are designed to rebuild, plump and lift, while those for the lower face streamline, slim and lift without adding bulk. This gives your face the right ratio: widest across the top of the cheekbones, neater and slimmer across the jaw. Ageing faces tend to be wider across the lower part of the face, due to the effect of gravity on sagging muscles. Faceworks restores the balance and turns the clock back. Lines and wrinkles reduce in spread and depth and you'll find that future wrinkling is minimised. A toned face that doesn't sag helps to prevent new lines from forming.

Every sign of ageing in the face has been matched with an exercise to work the muscles where they appear. For example; on the brows, ageing causes the brow arch to flatten and the whole brow drops. The result is low eyebrows and baggy, sagging top eyelids and folds at the outer eye corner. The Eyebrow Lift and Eye Toner Two lift the drooping brows by rebuilding the frontalis and corrugator supercilii muscles. This raises the brows up, gives a beautiful arch, lifts sagging on the lid, opens the eye and erases frown ridges and outer eye folds. No skin product can do this for you. Your body's ability to regenerate itself is the perfect beauty treatment.

Your Facial Muscles

Of the 630+ muscles in the human body, approximately 53 are found in the face. The true number varies, not all of us have every single muscle possible. The essential muscles to produce facial expression are always present; the non-essential ones can be a few short of the full set, which goes some way to explain why some people have less movement in their faces than others, or why one side of the face may move differently to the other.

Diagram 1: Superficial and Deep Facial Muscle Layers

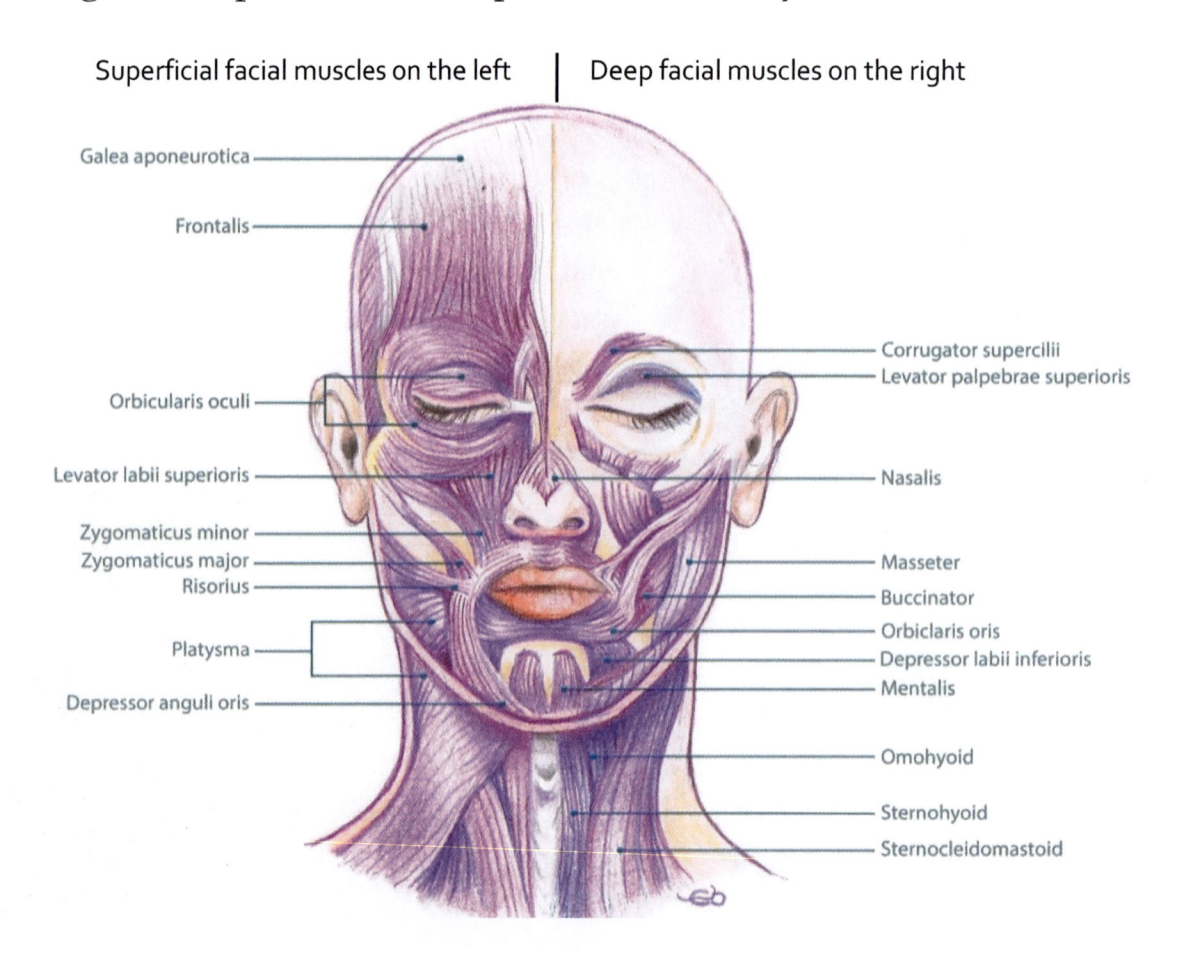

Facial muscles are part of our skeletal muscle system. Skeletal muscles move our bones and facial skin by contracting and relaxing, and we move them voluntarily.

There are two other types of muscles in the human body: cardiac muscle in the heart, and smooth muscle in internal organs. Both cardiac and smooth muscles are involuntary and work without our conscious thought.

Diagram 2: Superficial Facial Muscle Layer, Lateral View

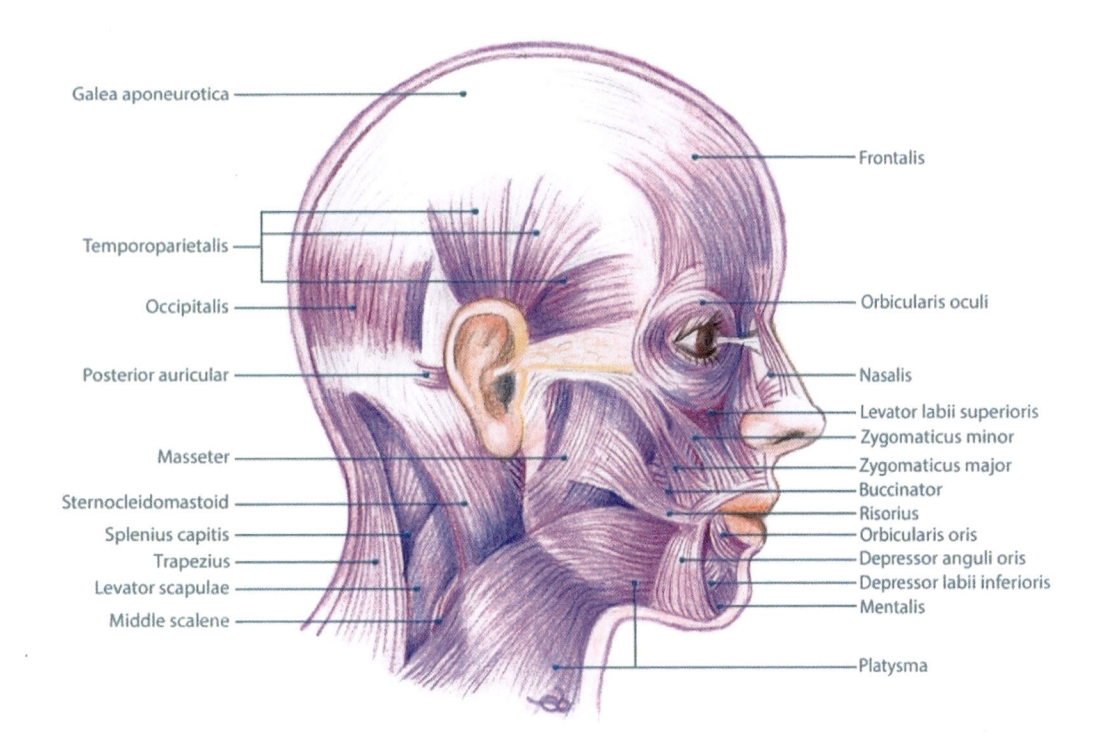

Humans and apes have specially adapted facial muscles. They enable us to communicate in far more sophisticated ways than other animals. These special muscles are attached at one end to the facial bones and insert into the base layers of the dermis: the skin. So we talk, laugh, frown and make all our facial expressions because of the muscles that move the skin.

This specialised ability makes a natural facelift possible. When we work the muscles of the face in specific ways, they get fitter and stronger. They tone up. They lift. And because the muscles are attached to the skin, it lifts too.

Diagram 3: Deep Facial Muscle Layer, Lateral View

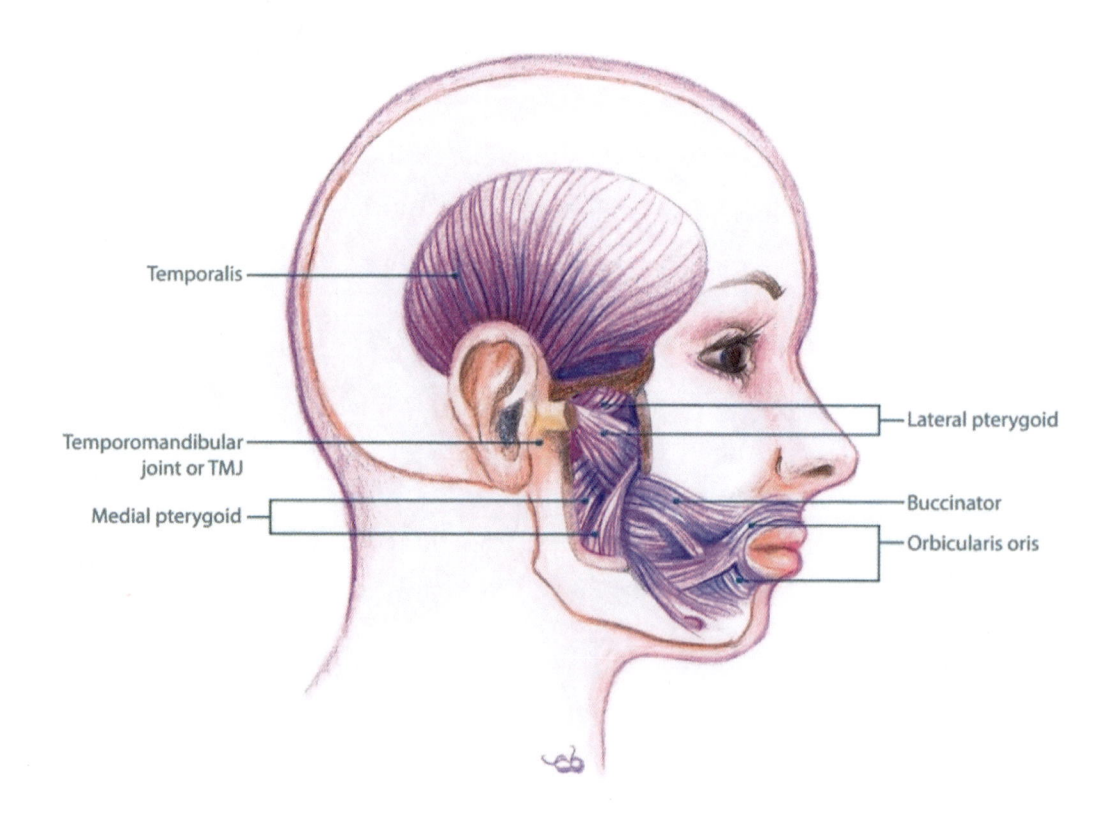

Muscles: the Body's Movers and Shakers

Skeletal muscle tissue is made up of groups of specialised elastic fibres; each powered by a nerve and bound together in bundles. The bundles are covered by connective tissues called the fascia which extend at each end into tendons to anchor the muscle to bones or other structures: facial muscles are attached to the facial bones and the dermis, and they enable movement.

Oxygen, nutrients and waste products are carried to and from the muscle by blood vessels. Lymph fluid collects waste products and micro-organisms for filtration through the lymph system.

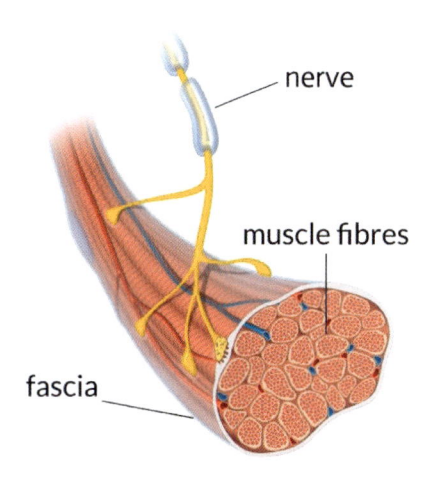

Muscles are incredible. They move everything within the body: blood through the heart (cardiac muscle), air through the lungs and the food we eat through the digestive tract (smooth muscle). Muscles are capable of great force, or the gentlest touch. Just one movement of your hand requires a synchronised action of nerve impulses and many muscles to produce a smooth, coordinated and precise result, yet all this can happen in a fraction of a second. Muscles contain fast-firing fibres and slow-firing fibres, and generate energy by either aerobic or anaerobic respiration. Movement is a complicated physical process!

Even when our bodies are relaxed, they have 'resting tone': where a small number of muscle fibres remain in a contracted state. Actual physical movement occurs when a greater number of individual fibres within the muscle contracts. This causes the muscles to shorten, initiating a pull on the tendons at the ends of the muscle, which in turn moves the structures they are attached to. Our bones could not move without muscles.

Science has separated muscle contraction into two types: isometric: when muscles contract but the body does not move, e.g. holding a plate out, and isotonic: when muscles contract and move part of the body, e.g. lowering a plate to a table. Most movements; including the Faceworks exercises, are a combination of both isometric and isotonic contraction.

Muscles only work by pulling, so they have to work in groups. To initiate movement in one direction, one half of a pair of muscles contracts and pulls while the opposing muscle relaxes. To move the other way, the first muscle relaxes while the other contracts. For example, when you close your eye, the orbicularis oculi around the eye contracts to close the lids and the levator palpebrae superioris on the top lid relaxes. The eye is opened as the levator muscle contracts and lifts the top lid, while the orbicularis oculi around the eye relaxes.

All facial muscles are served by the 7th cranial nerve, apart from the muscle that covers the top of the scalp: the levator palpebrae superioris, which is innervated by the 3rd cranial nerve.

How Exercise Rebuilds Your Facial Muscles

When muscles are worked regularly, they increase in size. The tiny myofibrils that make up each muscle fibre grow bigger and nerve impulses get stronger. Research has shown that people in their 80s and over benefit from regular exercise: it's never too late!

Faceworks uses gentle strength training to improve the fitness of facial muscles, without overbuilding them. As the muscles respond to the exercises, the nerve impulses that make the fibres contract become stronger. Each time you work out, more nerves answer the call and more fibres respond. With frequent exercise the resting tone of the facial muscles increases and they become 'tighter' and firmer. It has a huge impact on the look and feel of the face.

The size and shape of muscles is governed by the natural regeneration process. We're not talking about bulking muscle up; as in body building, but the ordinary ability to replace tissue. Muscles grow by a process of damage and repair, though not the kind of damage you would be aware of. Exercise causes microscopic damage to the muscle fibres. The tiny tears in the muscle stimulate the body's natural repair process: protein, hormones and nutrients combine to build bigger fibres that are able to cope with the increased workload.

If the workload decreases, so does the size of the muscles. The proteins in the fibres are broken down into amino acids and used elsewhere. The muscles return to their old size and shape, and eventually the resting tone decreases and the tissues slacken.

Healthy, fit muscles have a higher resting tone, a shorter, more compact shape and the strength to respond to demand more completely. Smaller, firmer and tighter muscles produce the facelift. Facial contours are defined, smoothed and rejuvenated.

Skin: the Body's Largest Organ

Anatomy of the Skin

The two major layers of the skin are the epidermis and the dermis. The epidermis at the top is divided into 4 levels: these top layers have no blood supply and are constantly shed as new cells move up through the epidermal layers. The deepest layer of the epidermis: the stratum basale, is where new living skin cells are made. Here too is melanin which gives skin its' natural colour. Skin cells take around 28 days to move up from the stratum basale to the surface of the skin, gradually dying as they migrate upwards.

The second major layer is the dermis. It is characterised by dense connective tissue, bundles of collagen fibres, elastin, blood and lymph vessels, nerves, sweat glands, sebaceous glands and hair follicles.

Underneath the dermis is the hypodermis or subcutaneous layer that attaches the skin to underlying tissues such as organs or muscles. This layer is bursting with fat cells and large blood vessels that supply nutrients to the skin. It's the quantity of fat cells in this layer that cushions skin in young faces, and unfortunately the fat gradually shifts and reduces as we get older.

The elastic fibres we hear so much about in relation to ageing are collagen, elastic, and reticular fibres. They are found in most types of connective tissue in the body, and play a vital role by maintaining strength and flexibility.

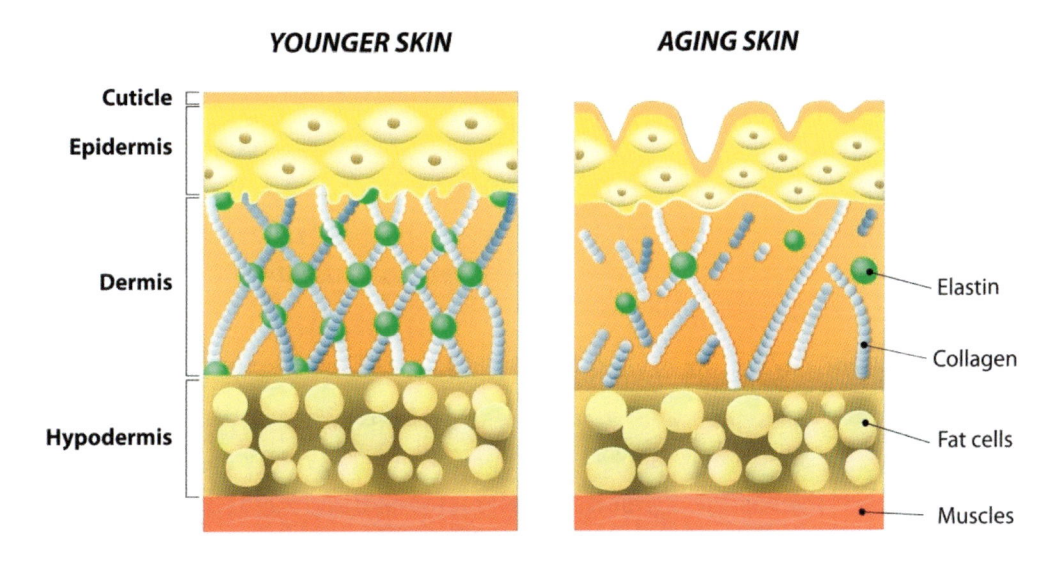

Our skin is the largest organ. It's the first to suffer when nutrition and water are in short supply and the last to benefit. Both wound healing and infection increase the need for good nutrition. When our bodies are fighting off illness, nutrients that would normally be available for repair are used up by the immune system for defence. You'll notice the tendency for your skin to look dry or dull when you have a cold, for example. If skin is damaged, healing requires protein and vitamins: most notably Vitamin C. A good diet and adequate hydration is vital to keep skin looking young and fresh.

Water is a great beauty treatment! Few of us drink enough or drink at the right times. To calculate how much water you should drink per day, find out what your weight is in pounds. Divide this amount by 3, the answer is the amount you should drink in fluid ounces, e.g. 180lbs divided by 3 gives 60 fl.ozs. of water. Try to drink away from meal times too: water dilutes digestive juices which can lead to indigestion or heartburn.

How Facial Exercise Transforms Your Skin

One of the great surprises when I developed Faceworks was the effect the exercises had on the skin. I had expected that the face would rebuild and change most, and the skin only slightly. How wrong I was! Let's look at the effects of exercise on your skin.

For most of us any exertion is immediately visible: even if we don't break into a sweat, we go red in the face. That glow is due to the expansion of the tiny blood capillaries; they are closer to the surface of the skin on your face than anywhere else in your body. Blood flow increases if the body works harder to bring oxygen and nutrition to the cells. The wastes are removed faster too: debris, excess fluid, free radicals and toxins are carried away for filtering through the liver and disposal via the kidneys or bowel.

Facial exercise is great news for your skin. Faces literally bloom in a way that's impossible with skin creams alone. Blood supply improves, bringing valuable nutrients that boost the production and quality of skin cells. Vitamin C, for example is absolutely vital for the formation and maintenance of collagen. The increase in blood supply also reduces potential damage from free radicals, chemicals and bacteria. Finally, excess fluid in the tissues is removed swiftly by the lymph fluid, reducing puffiness.

Both our research; and testimonials from people who use Faceworks, show the program has a beneficial effect on skin problems. In our client trial before Faceworks was launched, there were a number of skin abnormalities: spots, blackheads, T-zone greasiness, redness and dryness. All improved over the course of 12 weeks: to the delight of the test subjects. I thought the increase in circulation would be a secondary benefit when I began Faceworks, but it proved to bring as many improvements to the skin as to the muscles underneath.

A Note on Cosmetic Surgery

From the e-mails we get coming in from the website, the number one reason that prevents people from going through with surgery is the fear of things going wrong. Keeping the face you know is often better than letting a surgeon play God with your looks.

There is currently no legislation or regulating body for the less invasive procedures that include Botox and injectable fillers. Hopefully, in the near future this will change and there will be tighter regulations on the industry. In the UK, The Royal College of Surgeons recommends that "only licenced doctors, registered dentists and registered nurses should provide any cosmetic treatment". These guidelines include all laser and injectable treatments. The bottom line is, if you are considering any procedure, do your research and choose wisely.

Although I prefer a natural approach, I am not against cosmetic surgery at all. When I noticed: at around 40, that I wasn't looking so great any more, I mentally pencilled in a facelift for my 50th birthday. The temptation to change the face we're born with is hard enough to resist even without age creeping in, in todays' airbrushed world. But I have shelved the plan to get that facelift; I don't feel that I need it.

If you decide to invest in surgery, discuss how best to reintroduce face exercises with your chosen surgeon.

The Ageing Face

It's a fact that exercise slows and reverses the ageing process in muscles: it's printed in black and white in my enormous anatomy and physiology text book. The strength and size of all our muscles declines as we age, unless physical activity intervenes. This process begins around the age of 30, though the evidence may not be physically noticeable until later.

For your face, the age-related loss of muscle is accompanied by gradual changes to the fatty layer underneath the skin. Mostly we think of fat as a bad thing to have, especially if you're under twenty and desperately trying to lose the chubbiness that childhood has left behind. But that fatty layer serves to cushion the skin, especially around delicate features of the face. Once it starts to disappear, your muscles have to take up the job. And if they're not in good shape, you're in trouble.

Facial muscles drop as time goes on, becoming longer, thinner and flatter. All the contours of the face lose their height as muscles give in to gravity: even the tip of the nose sags lower as the connective tissues relax. This tilting down of everything that used to tilt up makes faces look tired, not to mention sad and unhappy. Consequently they look less interesting. We often think that lines and wrinkles are the culprit, but in my opinion there is nothing more ageing than a drooping face.

The bones of the face are also affected by ageing. The demineralisation of facial bones is most noticeable in the jaw and cheekbones: faces literally shrink. Bone is living tissue, constantly being absorbed and replaced according to the changing needs of the body. Any activity that requires stronger muscles builds stronger bones, while inactivity causes bone resorption. If you don't use it, you lose it! As bone mass increases with exercise, it may be that facial strength training with programs such as Faceworks may prevent age-related bone demineralisation in the face. At present this remains a theory, it will be interesting to see if my theory is correct in years to come.

So although you may complain about your wrinkles, it's actually the structure underneath that's making you look old and tired. Strong bones and plump muscles provide a firm structure and a deep cushion for the skin to rest on. The lost fatty layer isn't replaceable (unless you want to gain weight generally), but those out of shape muscles are capable of filling the space it used to occupy.

For skin, the ageing process is most noticeable where it is exposed to sunlight. Age slows the speed of cell renewal, and blood supply becomes less efficient. All the fibres responsible for keeping the skin plump and elastic change: becoming sparse, less elastic and disorganised. Skin becomes dryer, thinner and more prone to damage. Although the late forties is when ageing really starts to show; sun damage, smoking and poor nutrition can hasten the signs considerably.

New research is indicating that free radical activity in the body could be the biggest reason that skin ages. The natural process of cell oxidation creates free radicals, which damage healthy cells. Poor nutrition, smoking, illness and ageing are all known to increase the free radical load.

Our bodies are made up of cells, which in turn are made up of molecules. Molecules are like microscopic planets: each atom in the centre has even pairs of electrons orbiting around it, held in place by chemical bonds. If one electron is lost; leaving an odd number in orbit, the molecule becomes unbalanced and unstable. This is a free radical. If there are insufficient antioxidant vitamins circulating in the body to 'defuse' the free radical, it steals an electron from another body cell to re-stabilise itself. This initiates a cascade of damage within the cell, potentially causing cell death. Antioxidants however; stay stable even if they give up one of their electrons, so free radical damage is halted by them. Scientists theorise that if there are enough antioxidants circulating in the body to prevent free radicals from attacking other cells, ageing will progress at a slower rate. Of course this is not just beneficial for the face: your whole body constantly relies on nutrition to defuse free radicals.

Ageing Timeline

Without intervention from face exercise and effective preventative skincare, the skin and the supporting tissues gradually change as we grow older. Thankfully, we're no longer living in a time when a woman was 'old' at 40, but the signs of age continue to trace across our faces unless we're exceptionally careful to preserve what we have:

20s

The skin is firm and smooth with few lines. Collagen, elastic and reticular fibres are in abundance in the dermis and subcutaneous layers, providing elasticity. Cell turnover is at its' peak with a constant sloughing of dead skin cells: skin is consequently bright and luminous. The lipid layer and subcutaneous fat pads under the dermis plump the skin, softening facial contours. The only usual causes of epidermal degradation in this age group are sun damage, smoking, poor nutrition and air pollution.

30s

Although the complexion is still rosy and bright, the delicate skin around the eyes begins to sag. Habitual expressions leave permanent fine lines across the forehead, between the brows and at the eye corners. The lipid layer begins to reduce. By the late 30s, muscles have started to lengthen and the cheeks look flatter. The mouth corners settle lower and lines between the mouth and nose corners become more noticeable. The demands of a career and possibly children can mean that skin nourishing nutrition is the last thing on your 'essentials' list, and skin can age faster than it should for this age group.

40s

Ageing signs are more widespread. The face looks generally tired as muscles continue their downward journey. Expression lines are deeper, and skin suffers from slowing cell production and the change in elasticity. The general condition of the skin is drier, and it may look patchy or dull. The fatty layer under the dermis continues to shrink, causing under eye hollows and looser skin. Hooded lids and eye bags are common. The lower facial height gets shorter as the soft tissues relax, and the jawline softens.

50s

Facial hair growth patterns alter with the change in hormones brought about by the menopause. Eyebrows can become patchy and drop lower. Delicate eye skin above the top lid falls lower over the lid and at the outer eye corner. The nose tip drops and vertical lines appear above and below the lips. Facial lines become entrenched as tissues sag, creating folds around the eyes, nose and mouth. For some women the menopause accounts for rapid changes to the quality of the skin, not just for the face but over the whole body. The elasticity of skin is reduced as collagen and other fibres become thicker and less responsive, the skin looks more uneven with a network of fine lines. The contours around the chin and jaw are not as well defined, jowls and scalloping around the chin masks the true face shape.

60s, 70s and beyond

Skin folds and lines continue to deepen. The facial contours are disturbed as the underlying tissues reduce and shrink, with facial muscles losing 40% of their mass at time goes on. Remaining subcutaneous fat pads create an uneven surface as they settle lower, characterised by eye bags, gaunt upper cheeks, heaviness around the mouth and further softening of the jawline. Bone structure changes, most notably the eye orbit enlarges and both upper and lower jaws shrink. Teeth may become loose. The lips lose their supporting structure and thin down, more vertical lip lines may appear. Cartilage in the ears and nose soften and both look longer. The weight of slack muscles in the cheek creates heaviness around the lower face and jaw. The face shape alters considerably, becoming flatter and longer.

The Development of Faceworks

The seed of an idea for a face exercise program came into my head while I was studying for my Anatomy and Physiology Diploma in 2001. I wondered that; if muscles developed and regenerated in the way my textbooks said, was it possible to use exercise as a viable alternative to cosmetic surgery? At the time, I had plenty to occupy me after qualifying in my chosen therapies of Kinesiology and Reiki, setting up my small practice and family life, and I didn't revisit the idea for some time.

About four years later, I was working with a client. She was a regular and we had addressed her nutritional needs, balanced her body and gone through the issues she wanted to work with over a period of a couple of months. It often happens that the health concern that brings a client through the door is a symptom, and the body reveals the core issue: the real cause of the problem, after the symptoms are resolved. It's a lot like the layers of an onion, the body brings out what it needs to work through in its' own time. Complementary therapies work with the body to address symptoms as they appear, while working towards and hopefully resolving the core issue. These core issues are often due in whole or in part, to an emotional trigger that prevents us from enjoying our lives and living to our fullest potential.

We had come to the end of her session and were talking through the treatment, when she sighed heavily and said: "I want to be young and beautiful again". That was her core issue and right then, my therapies didn't have an answer. If ever I needed a reason to explore my idea; I had it.

That sentence gave me the impetus for some serious investigation. Clients often asked me if I could make them look as good as they felt after their treatment, now I had a challenge. When Faceworks became a reality three years later, that lady was one of the first people to learn the exercises.

Research

So what kind of rejuvenating therapy would work? From my training, I knew that rebuilding the facial muscles was potentially the best option for a natural facelift. But before I went any further, I looked at every natural method I could think of to reduce the signs of ageing and keep the face looking healthy. As I researched, it became ever more obvious that the failing of the structure under the skin was to blame for looking old. The changes to and the loss of muscle didn't provide the skin enough support. It didn't matter how many creams were put on the surface, none of them could go deep enough to get to the source of the problem.

I have always been fascinated by how the body works. For my new research, it was a good interest to have! While I'd learned the about health problems associated with some facial and scalp muscles in Kinesiology, I put myself back into study to research the origin, insertion and action of the rest of the facial muscles. I designed about 30 exercises to work different areas of the face in a variety of ways. Introducing a focus point for each exercise, I used slight variations in position to work the facial muscles comprehensively and improve the strength and condition quickly. After testing them individually (which took quite a while) I put the most effective into a set and began doing them 5 times a week at my dressing table mirror. My flat, drooping 45 year old face was the perfect guinea-pig. As I wanted to get an unbiased reaction, I didn't tell my family what I was doing. After a month I asked them if they noticed any difference. All I told them was that I had changed my skincare regime. "More smiley", "Less tired-looking" and "Better, but not sure how", were the comments cautiously returned.

People began to tell me that I looked well. My children said that I didn't look cross all the time because my frown lines had disappeared. As my face changed, I discovered a new confidence in myself. Getting out of bed in the morning was suddenly something to look forward to.

After three months of working my face, I had surprise reaction to the 'new me'. The downside of doing anything gradually: like going to the gym or losing weight, is that it's only people who don't see you every day who get the full impact. I had no idea how different I looked until we happened to see some friends one evening. At first I thought I had spinach in my teeth. When my friend dragged me into a corner I thought I had upset her, but it was because she wanted to know what on earth I'd been doing: she thought I'd had surgery.

I knew beyond doubt that the exercises worked: and it was time for a bigger trial. I am indebted to the ladies and colleagues who worked with me to test the exercises fully. The age range was from early 30s to mid-50s, with a variety of skin types and individual needs. In all cases, the exercises produced measurable changes to facial structure and skin condition. An increase in self-confidence progressed in tandem with physical improvement.

Official Recognition

Faceworks was approved as a new therapy by the Complementary Therapists' Association (CThA) in the UK in 2008. Gaining official recognition enables a modality to be offered to the public, so potential clients are assured that the therapy meets professional standards. Faceworks is the only facial exercise program to achieve this status.

From Small Acorns

My only ambition with Faceworks was to teach it to clients in my practice. But my husband said I looked so different and he thought I should do more with it: "Like put it on the internet". In 2005, social media was in its' infancy. YouTube had only just launched, and using video on the internet was a new phenomenon. It seemed an odd direction to go in, but the global recession at the time was biting and I thought it would be wise to broaden my reach. It was a huge learning curve.

I found a company who made films for TV and industry to do the videos. Quadrillion: based in Marlow, were great, to their credit they never raised an eyebrow at my weird request to film face exercises. It took me months to drum up the courage to do the shoot and have a production crew watch and film while I went through the exercises, but eventually I ran out of excuses. With my husband giggling like an idiot while he 'helpfully' read my script off camera, we got the films done in one take.

The first website went live in 2007, with just one workout and a basic service. As the internet evolved and people told us how they wanted to use the exercises, the program developed into a variety of workouts. Over the years, despite continued research I have not discovered any exercises that work better; or more completely, than the originals.

Technology continuously opens up new possibilities, and keeping abreast of the enormous changes in the way we share information is exciting and challenging. Most recently, the YouTube videos have seen an exponential rise in views with over a million new hits in just 3 weeks.

Throughout this time, the response to the exercises remains the same: people are surprised and delighted that they work, and they're incredulous that they can achieve the changes for themselves.

Postscript

Looking good changes how people feel about themselves. It is a powerful feeling, and it's not an exaggeration to say that it opens life up to new possibilities: new ways of being.

Enjoy the new way of being you.

We'd love to hear your experience with Faceworks. Please review the book on Amazon or send your comments by e-mail to helpdesk@faceworks.co.uk.

Glossary of Terms

Asana: A yoga position or posture.

Crow's feet: Permanent lines that fan out from the outside corner of the eyes, usually made by facial expressions such as smiling or laughing.

Cupid's bow: The centre of the upper lip that is said to be shaped like a cupid's bow, formed by the two points of the upper lip and the dip in between. When the lips thin with age, the Cupid's bow becomes shallower.

Circulation: Usually refers to the flow of blood or lymph around the body. Blood pumped by the heart through the arteries supplies oxygen and nutrition to cells. Waste products and carbon dioxide are removed by the veins and lymph.

Dermis: The living layer of skin under the epidermis, containing both blood supply and nerves.

Endocrine glands: specialised glands that secrete hormones into the blood to keep the body functioning properly. Hormones control processes such as digestion, metabolism, reproduction and growth.

Epidermis: The layer of skin that we can see. It consists of 5 layers that are gradually replaced from below. There is no blood supply in this layer and the cells die as they move up to the surface.

Eye bags: Puffy, swollen tissue under the skin, usually below the lower eye lid. They may contain excess fluid (oedema) and/or fat and may be a different colour to the surrounding skin.

Eye hollows: A dip or hollow below the lower lids, caused by the decline in the fat pad under the eye and the loosening of the cheek muscles. Also caused by age related bone loss around the orbit of the eye (eye socket).

Frown furrows: Vertical grooves between the eyebrows, caused by frowning and facial expression and gradual slackening of the muscles on the brow ridge. Sometimes called the 'Number 11's'.

Hooded eyes: Sagging skin between the eyebrows and the eyelid that covers the top lid.

Hyoid: The hyoid bone is a horseshoe-shaped bone in the front of the neck that enables the tongue to move and assists in swallowing. The many muscles around the hyoid bone keep it in position level with bottom of the lower jaw.

Jowls: pouch-shaped sagging skin either side of the mouth that may drop below the line of the jaw.

Larynx: An organ in the front of the neck that contains the voice box. The Larynx is the top part of the tube that runs from behind the tongue to the trachea to enable respiration (breathing).

Lipid layer: See 'subcutaneous layer'

Lymph: The lymphatic system supports blood circulation and protects the body against infection. Lymph fluid circulates in the body and removes waste products and invading micro-organisms by filtration through lymph nodes and the Spleen.

Marionette lines: Lines that run from the outer corners of the mouth down to the bottom of the chin. They resemble the lines on puppets (marionettes) and ventriloquists' dolls that enable the puppet to open its' mouth.

Muscles: Muscles are groups of tissue that are attached to other parts of the body to enable movement. Muscle fibres contract and change shape, so moving the structures they are attached to.

Naso-labial folds: Folds and creases that run from the bottom corner of the nose out to the corners of the mouth. They are caused by softening of the cheek muscles and loose skin.

Neck vertebrae: The bones in the upper spine, i.e. the neck, usually called the cervical vertebrae.

Parathyroid glands: Paired endocrine glands in the neck, responsible for maintaining calcium in the circulation. They are located on the thyroid glands.

Scalloping: Softened, sagging skin along the line of the jaw that forms an uneven line.

Subcutaneous layer: The layer of tissue directly under the dermis. It consists primarily of loose connective tissue and fat cells, plus large blood vessels and nerves.

Tear troughs: Small, trough-like depressions that can be seen below the inner corners of the eyes and which tears run along on their exit from the eye. They may be darker than the surrounding skin.

Temporo-mandibular joint: The main jaw joint that attaches the lower jaw to the skull. It can be found directly below the ears and is a common site of tension-related pain. It is one of the most complicated joints in the body.

Trachea: More commonly known as the wind-pipe, it runs down the front of the neck from the larynx into the chest where it divides into two branches and continues to the lungs.

Thyroid glands: Paired endocrine glands on the front of the neck that control tissue metabolism and metabolic rate.

Vertical lip lines: Lines that form on the edge of the lips, caused by thinning of the lips due to age.

Acknowledgements

Thanks to Immortaleye Photography for all the exercise photos, advice and expertise.

Thanks to Joe Bartlett for taking care of all the technical and formatting work for this book that was too complicated for my pre-computer age brain to deal with.

Thanks to my daughter, Leah for proof-reading and suggestions. I resisted your critique that the book needed some diagrams but I enjoyed doing the artwork and the book is so much better for them.

Lastly, thanks to my irrepressible husband: Graham, for your enthusiasm, support and crazy off the wall ideas that always work.

And finally, thanks to you for knocking age into the stratosphere and proving that looking fabulous isn't the sole preserve of the under 30s.

Bibliography and Resources

Tortora and Grabowski. Principles of Anatomy and Physiology, 9th Edition. Wiley & Sons. Inc

Mary. E. Barasi BA, BSc, Msc. Human Nutrition, A Health Perspective, Second Edition. Hodder Arnold.

Louise Tucker, An Introductory Guide to Anatomy and Physiology, Holistic Therapy Books.

Patrick Holford: New Optimum Nutrition Bible, Piatkus

Brian H. Butler, Kinesiology for Balanced Health, Volume One, Part II, T.A.S.K. Books

A. Lam, Kinesiology: A Compendium of Techniques, 2nd Edition, Green World Books

Dr. Brigid Waller, et al University of Portsmouth (2008, June 17). Learning From The Dead: What Facial Muscles Can Tell Us About Emotion. ScienceDaily

Richard Weil, Med CDE, How Muscles Work and How They Respond to Resistance Exercise, MedicineNet.com

Sydney Coleman, MD, Rajiv Grover BSc, MB BS, MD FRCS (Plast), Anatomy of the Aging Face: Volume Loss and Changes in 3-Dimensional Topography. Aesthetic Surgery Journal, Jan/Feb 2006

Complimentary Therapists' Association: https://www.ctha.com

ITEC: http://www.itecworld.co.uk

Kinesiology Association, Registered Charity Number 299306
https://www.kinesiologyassociation.org

Greater Medical Council (UK): http://www.gmc-uk.org

Printed in Great Britain
by Amazon